Praise for

Solution to Type 2 Diabetes

"Ms. Tessmer's book **Your Nutrition Solution to Type 2 Diabetes** is right on! As a diabetes educator she has covered the important lessons of diabetes self-management. I would highly recommend this book to my patients who have been diagnosed with diabetes. She uses a friendly dialog in her writing that made me feel like I was talking to a friend who was there to help me, if I were a person diagnosed with diabetes."

—Hope Williams, RD, CDE

"Another great, helpful diet guide by renowned nutritionist Kim Tessmer! Explains type 2 diabetes and its most vital treatment strategy—diet—in an easy-to-understand way! Dispels many popular diabetic diet myths as well. Full of realistic, helpful food suggestions—a great resource for my patients!"

—Karyn Lyn Abdallah, MD

"I like the nutrition tidbit sections. I think this is a good resource for people who are newly diagnosed and have lots of questions about the disease."

—Joyce Giammattei, DrPH, RD, CDE

"Have you or a loved one been diagnosed with type 2 diabetes? You've come to the right place! In this comprehensive guide, Kim decodes type 2 diabetes step by step and answers your questions about the disease, diet, medications, and supplements. You will be empowered with the knowledge and tools you need to make healthy lifestyle changes and the confidence to implement your nutrition solution."

—Michaela Ballmann, MS, RD, CLT, Founder, Wholify

"The meal ideas and Nutrition Solution Tidbits in this book will be a great help to take the confusion and frustration out of eating healthier with type 2 diabetes!"

—Karen Marschel, RDN, LD, CDE, KM, Nutrition Consulting, Inc.

your nutrition
SOLUTION
to
TYPE 2 DIABETES

a meal-based plan to
help manage diabetes

kimberly a. tessmer, RDN, LD

New Page Books
a division of The Career Press, Inc.
Pompton Plains, N.J.

Your Nutrition Solution to Type 2 Diabetes
Edited and Typeset by Kara Kumpel
Cover design by Joanna Williams
Printed in the U.S.A.

To order this title, please call toll-free 1-800-CAREER-1 (NJ and Canada: 201-848-0310) to order using VISA or MasterCard, or for further infor-mation on books from Career Press.

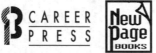

The Career Press, Inc.
220 West Parkway, Unit 12
Pompton Plains, NJ 07444
www.careerpress.com
www.newpagebooks.com

Library of Congress Cataloging-in-Publication Data
Tessmer, Kimberly A.
    Your nutrition solution to Type 2 diabetes : a meal-based plan to help manage diabetes / by Kimberly Tessmer, RD, LD.
        pages cm
    Includes index.
    Summary: "The correct diet plan can be the key to lowering or even eliminating the need for prescription medications and living a life without the worry of medical complications due to type 2 diabetes. This book will give you the tools and meal plans to put you on the right path"-- Provided by publisher.
        ISBN 978-1-60163-325-5 (paperback) -- ISBN 978-1-60163-446-7 (ebook) 1. Non-insulin-dependent diabetes--Nutritional aspects--Popular works. 2. Non-insulin-dependent diabetes--Diet therapy--Recipes. I. Title.

RC662.18.T44 2014
641.5'6314--dc23

2014014337

Dedication

I dedicate this book to all the people who deal daily with type 2 diabetes. My hope is that this book is able to help you relieve the fear and frustration that goes along with being diagnosed with type 2 diabetes, and that it will empower you to make the necessary changes you need to start feeling better and manage your diabetes for a lifetime.

As always, I also dedicate this book to my dad and to my late mom, whom I miss dearly. I am so thankful for the gift they passed on to me for helping others. That is what gives me my passion to be a dietitian and help others deal with their struggles.

Acknowledgments

A loving thank-you to my wonderful husband, Greg, who works so hard, which allows me to do what I love, and to my daughter, Tori, who is always patient and gives Mommy the time to do her writing. I would like to thank all of my fellow RDs who gave me their expert input and advice on this subject. A special thank-you to the dietitians who took the time to review my book and provide endorsements.

Disclaimer

At the time this book was written, all information in this book was believed by the author to be correct and accurate. Information on type 2 diabetes changes frequently as more research is being completed. Always keep yourself up to date by reading reputable and current publications and speaking with your healthcare provider. The author shall have no liability of any kind for damages of any nature, however caused. The author will not accept any responsibility for any omissions, misinterpretations, or misstatements that may exist within this book. The author does not endorse any product or company listed in this book. Always consult with your healthcare provider for medical advice as well as recommendations on any type of supplement or herbal supplement you plan on taking. The author is not engaged in rendering medical services, and this book should not be construed as medical advice, nor should it take the place of being properly diagnosed and monitored by your regular healthcare provider.

contents

introduction

If you have been diagnosed with diabetes, you already know there is more than one form of the disease and that they vastly differ. Type 2 diabetes is the most common form, and, thankfully, it's is also the one that can, for the most part, be properly managed with nutritional intervention. Unfortunately, the prevalence of type 2 diabetes continues to increase. In fact, according to the American Diabetes Association, the prevalence of diagnosed diabetes increased by 128 percent from the years 1988 to 2008, and in the years since it has continued to rise. If this trend continues, the Association predicts that 1 in 3 American adults will have diabetes by 2050, with the majority of those cases being type 2 diabetes. A whopping 25.8 million—yes, that is *million*—people in the United States are currently affected by some form of diabetes. That's 8.3 percent of all adults and children in the United States. Of these 25.8 million people, 18.8 million are diagnosed cases and 7 million are undiagnosed—and what is not diagnosed cannot be treated! Type 2 diabetes accounts for 90 to 95 percent of all these cases. In U.S. adults aged 65 and older, 10.9 million or 26.9 percent have diabetes, and 215,000 people under the age of 20 have diabetes. Sadly, type 2 diabetes, once referred to as "adult onset" diabetes, is no longer an adult-only disease, and is increasingly being found in children and teens. In addition to all of these diagnosed and undiagnosed cases of diabetes are countless numbers of people who have *prediabetes*, a condition that puts them at higher risk of developing type 2 diabetes in the future. I think you get the idea that diabetes is an enormous and ongoing problem in our population, and one that touches people of all ages.

The difficult part for people with type 2 diabetes is that treatment is very individualized and can differ greatly from one person to the next. Each individual's treatment plan will vary depending on blood sugar levels and the severity of his or her disease. The goal for people with type 2 diabetes is to create normal and consistent blood sugar levels, which involves individualized eating patterns, exercise, and, for some, medications or insulin. Diabetes can be a complicated disease, but here's the good news:

- That there *is* help out there.
- Type 2 diabetes *can* be managed.

This book will provide you with all the tools you need to better understand and manage your disease and to reach the ultimate goal of living a happy, healthy life with diabetes. Although nutritional intake is a huge part of managing type 2 diabetes, I also share in this book other essential aspects of your lifestyle that will help you to control your blood sugar, including body weight, exercise, and stress release. Because not all people with type 2 diabetics are created equal, you will find that this book will provide you with information on more than one way to handle eating. Once you have all the facts, you can more easily discuss with your doctor the best course of action for you. Seeking one-on-one help from a registered dietitian nutritionist (RDN) and/or a certified diabetes educator (CDE) is also highly recommended if you have been diagnosed with diabetes. This book will act as an aide to enlighten you on the subject before you speak with your doctor and other healthcare providers and provide you with essential information at your fingertips whenever you need it. Now is the time to take charge of your own health. This book is *your* nutrition solution to type 2 diabetes!

chapter 1

your questions about type 2 diabetes—answered

You just heard the news from your doctor: you have type 2 diabetes. Now what? What does that mean? Naturally you have loads of important questions swirling around in your head. Here are some common questions and their answers to help you sort through all of the information surrounding type 2 diabetes. Once you have a better understanding of the hows, whats, and whys of diabetes, you will be ready to dive right into the nutrition and lifestyle changes you need to make to feel better and lower your risk for serious health complications in the future. This is your perfect starting point!

What is diabetes?

Diabetes, or diabetes mellitus, is a group of metabolic disorders in which the body is unable to produce any or enough insulin and/or to use it properly. This results in levels of blood glucose (sugar) rising higher than normal levels. Glucose in your blood comes from the digestion of carbohydrates and is an essential form of sugar that your body uses for energy. In addition, the liver both stores and produces glucose depending on your body's needs. However, sometimes too much of a good thing can be harmful; too much glucose or blood sugar over time can do plenty of damage to your body.

What is insulin?

Insulin is a hormone produced by beta cells in the pancreas and released into the bloodstream. It plays a major role in metabolism, or the way the body uses digested foods for energy. Insulin helps cells in the body to absorb glucose and use it and/or store it as energy for future use. In a healthy person, the actions of insulin helps blood glucose levels to remain in the normal range.

What is insulin resistance?

Insulin resistance happens when the body has a problem using insulin effectively. With insulin resistance, cells within the muscles, fat, and liver do not respond properly to insulin and therefore are not able to absorb glucose from the blood-stream. This results in the body needing higher levels of insulin for the glucose to enter the cells. The pancreas tries to keep up with the increased demand by producing more, but in time fails to do so, and that increases the risk for prediabetes and type 2 diabetes. Although insulin resistance is never the sole cause of type 2 diabetes, it often increases the risk by placing a high demand on the beta cells in the pancreas that produce insulin. Most people don't even know they have insulin resistance until they end up with prediabetes and/or type 2 diabetes. If a person is aware he has insulin resistance he is often able to prevent or delay type 2 diabetes by making the necessary diet and lifestyle changes.

What does it mean if you have prediabetes?

Prediabetes simply means that your blood sugar levels are higher than normal but not high enough to yet be diagnosed with type 2 diabetes. Once the beta cells can no longer produce enough insulin to conquer the condition of insulin resistance, blood glucose levels rise to an abnormal level. Before people develop type 2 diabetes they almost always have prediabetes. Prediabetes is also referred to as *impaired glucose tolerance* (IGT) or *impaired fasting glucose* (IFG). People with prediabetes are at higher risk for many serious health issues, including heart disease and stroke. A whopping 35 percent of U.S. adults over 20 years of age and 50 percent of those over 65 years of age have prediabetes, which often occurs in people who already have insulin resistance. Once a person has prediabetes, the continuing failure of the beta cells to produce insulin can lead to type 2 diabetes, especially if diet and lifestyle changes are not made. Because there aren't many clear-cut symptoms, few of these people even know they have prediabetes.

Test results that indicate prediabetes include:

- ✳ An A1C level of 5.7 to 6.4 percent
- ✳ A fasting blood glucose level of 100 to 125 mg/dL (milligrams per deciliter)
- ✳ A 2-hour oral glucose tolerance test level of 140 to 199 mg/dL

Even if you are diagnosed with prediabetes, that in no way means you will automatically end up with type 2 diabetes. In fact, being diagnosed with prediabetes can be a blessing in disguise in that it gives you the chance to make eating and lifestyle changes now so that you do not end up with type 2 diabetes. Prediabetes is your warning sign that changes need to be made. If you have risk factors related to prediabetes you should be tested on a regular basis. The American Diabetes Association recommends blood glucose screening if you have any of the following risk factors for prediabetes:

- Are 45 years or older
- Are overweight, with a body mass index (BMI) above 25
- Are inactive (especially if you are also overweight)
- Have a parent or sibling with diabetes
- Have a family history of type 2 diabetes
- Are African American, Hispanic, American Indian, Asian American, or a Pacific Islander
- Have had gestational diabetes with a pregnancy or have given birth to a baby weighing more than 9 pounds
- Have a history of polycystic ovary syndrome (PCOS)
- Have high blood pressure
- Have high blood cholesterol levels, including a high-density lipoprotein (HDL), or "good" cholesterol, below 35 mg/dL, or triglyceride level above 250 mg/dL

Any of these risk factors will increase your risk for prediabetes. If you are screened and have normal blood sugar levels you will still need to be screened on a regular basis at your doctor's discretion. If you test positive for prediabetes, further testing may need to be done. Treatment will normally include eating a healthier diet, becoming more physically active, weight loss if needed, and medication if needed.

Your Nutrition Solution Tidbit: The American Diabetes Association states that you can cut your risk of moving from prediabetes to type 2 diabetes by 58 percent by losing just 7 percent of your body weight and exercising moderately 30 minutes a day, five days a week.

What is the difference between type 1 diabetes and type 2 diabetes?

There are several forms of diabetes, and they differ dramatically.

In **type 1 diabetes** (formerly known as *insulin-dependent diabetes* or *juvenile diabetes*), the body's immune system destroys the insulin-producing beta cells, resulting in a complete deficiency of insulin. In other words, in people with type 1 diabetes, the body produces absolutely no insulin. Normally when we eat food, the sugar (or glucose) stimulates our pancreas to release the right amount of insulin for whatever we ate. In people with type 1 diabetes, whose pancreas does not produce insulin, glucose does not move into the cells as it normally should because there is no insulin to do the job. What results is a buildup of blood glucose and high blood sugar levels. This can cause dehydration, weight loss, diabetic ketoacidosis (DKA), and damage to nerves, eyes, kidneys, and heart. Despite ongoing and active research, there currently is no cure for type 1 diabetes. It is a life-long disease. The treatment for type 1 diabetes includes intensive insulin therapy and continuous monitoring of blood sugar levels along with thorough meal planning and exercise.

The key to good health and a long life is keeping blood sugar at proper levels. All people with type 1 diabetes must use insulin as a life-saving method to control their blood sugar. If type 1 diabetes is not properly controlled a host of serious and life-threatening health issues can occur.

Type 1 diabetes normally occurs in people under the age of 20, but it can occur in older people as well. This form of diabetes is relatively uncommon and accounts for only about 5 percent of all people with diabetes. Although researchers are not completely sure what causes type 1 diabetes they do know that the condition can be genetic and can possibly be caused by exposure to certain viruses. Because type 1 diabetes is an auto-immune disease, it can occur along with other autoimmune disorders.

Your Nutrition Solution Tidbit: *Diabetic ketoacidosis* (DKA) occurs when the deficiency of insulin causes the energy-starved cells to break down fat cells. The breakdown of fat cells produces acidic chemicals called *ketones*, which can then be used for energy. Eventually these ketones begin to build up in the blood causing an increase in acidity. In the meantime, the liver continues to release sugar it has stored to help out but since the body cannot use this sugar without insulin, blood sugar levels continue to rise. This combination of high blood sugar, dehydration, and the buildup of acid is known as *ketoacidosis*, and it can be life-threatening if not treated immediately.

Type 2 diabetes is much different from type 1 diabetes and is the most common form of diabetes, affecting 90 to 95 percent of the almost 26 million people with diabetes. The big difference between type 1 diabetes and type 2 diabetes is that people with type 2 diabetes *do* make insulin in their bodies. The trouble in people with type 2 diabetes is that the pancreas either does not make *enough* insulin or the body does not use the insulin effectively. As we discussed, when there is not enough insulin or the body is not using insulin as it should, the glucose we get from the foods we eat cannot enter into the body's cells, and therefore these cells cannot perform their normal duties. High blood sugar is the outcome, which can do serious damage to the body in time. Another big difference between type 1 and type 2 diabetes is that a significant majority of people with type 2 diabetes can treat their condition with diet and exercise alone, though some may require oral medications or insulin in addition. Type 2 diabetes can be reversed in some with the right type of treatment and lifestyle changes and does not always have to be a life-long disease as type 1 diabetes is.

What is gestational diabetes?

One more form of diabetes to mention is gestational diabetes. This form of diabetes only affects pregnant women and is found in approximately 18 percent of all pregnancies. As with type 2 diabetes, insulin resistance and high blood sugar levels characterize gestational diabetes. Most pregnant women experience somewhat higher blood sugar levels, resulting from the hormonal changes that occur during pregnancy. During the last trimester of pregnancy these hormonal changes put women at the highest risk for gestational diabetes.

You have a higher risk of gestational diabetes if you:

- Had gestational diabetes with a previous pregnancy
- Previously gave birth to a baby weighing more than 9 pounds

- ⚮ Are older than 25 years of age
- ⚮ Are overweight before becoming pregnant
- ⚮ Have been diagnosed with prediabetes

Women who are at higher risk for gestational diabetes are usually screened as early as possible during their pregnancy and then again later in their pregnancy to confirm the diagnosis. For all other women, initial screening normally takes place between the 24th and 28th weeks of pregnancy. If not properly diagnosed and treated, this form of diabetes can affect the pregnancy and the baby's health. The good news is that gestational diabetes can be treated with the proper diet and exercise along with blood glucose monitoring and medication if needed. With gestational diabetes, blood sugar levels usually return to normal soon after the baby is born. However, if you develop gestational diabetes during your pregnancy it does put you at greater risk for developing type 2 diabetes in the future. If you experience gestational diabetes, the American Diabetes Association recommends getting screened for diabetes every three years.

What are normal blood sugar levels, and how are they tested?

Blood sugar is also known as blood glucose. Glucose comes from the foods we eat, specifically carbohydrates, and is our body's main source of energy. Normally, your blood glucose or blood sugar increases slightly after you eat. When blood sugar increases, your pancreas automatically releases insulin to keep levels from getting too high.

Before we can discuss what levels are normal, we have to introduce the tests used to determine those levels. There are several types of tests used to measure the level of blood sugar in the body:

- **Fasting Blood Sugar (FBS):** This test measures blood sugar after not eating for at least eight hours. FBS is often used as part of the diagnostic tool for prediabetes and diabetes.

- **2-hour Postprandial Blood Sugar**: This test measures blood sugar exactly two hours after eating a meal. This is usually not used as a diagnostic tool.

- **Random Blood Sugar (RBS):** This test measures blood sugar regardless of the timing of eating. RBS can be helpful because blood sugar levels in healthy people do not vary much throughout the day, so measurements that vary widely throughout the day can indicate a problem.

- **Oral Glucose Tolerance Test (OGTT):** This test is a series of blood sugar measurements that are taken at certain intervals after drinking a liquid that contains glucose. OGTT is commonly used to diagnose gestational diabetes in pregnant women as well as prediabetes and diabetes in other individuals.

The "normal" value ranges given for each test in the following list are considered only a guide. Ranges can vary from lab to lab, and your doctor will need to evaluate your results based on your health, age, and other factors to make a proper diagnosis.

- **Fasting Blood Sugar:** A normal range is between 70 and 100 mg/dL

- **2-hour Postprandial Blood Sugar:** A normal range is less than 140 mg/dL for people age 50 and younger, less than 150 mg/dL for people ages 50 to 60, and less than 160 mg/dL for people older than 60 years.

- **Random Blood Sugar:** Levels will vary depending on when you ate and how much you ate. A normal level is usually below 140 mg/dl.

⚄ **Oral Glucose Tolerance Test:** Using the 75-gram oral glucose tolerance test, a normal value for fasting is 70 to 100 mg/dl; after 1 hour it's less than 200 mg/dl, and after two hours it's less than 140 mg/dl.

Your Nutrition Solution Tidbit: Some people with type 2 diabetes need to not only be concerned about high blood sugar levels but low blood sugar, or *hypoglycemia*, as well. The American Diabetes Association states that there is a strong correlation between severe hypoglycemia and an increased risk of cardiovascular disease, including heart attack and stroke—another essential reason to closely monitor your blood sugar levels. Speak with your doctor if low blood sugar levels are a concern for you.

What is the A1C test?

The hemoglobin A1C test, also known as *HbA1C*, *glycated hemoglobin test*, or *glycohemoglobin*, is used to diagnose prediabetes, type 1 diabetes, and type 2 diabetes, as well as measure how well your diabetes or blood sugar is being controlled. The test provides an average of your blood sugar levels throughout a two- to three-month period, as opposed to your blood sugar level at one point in time, so it is a good indicator of whether changes to medication and/or lifestyle need to be made.

Hemoglobin is a protein in red blood cells that carries oxygen throughout our body. Glucose enters red blood cells and links up, or *glycates*, with hemoglobin. The more glucose there is in the blood the more hemoglobin becomes glycated. The A1C test measures what percentage of your hemoglobin is coated with glucose (glycated). The higher your A1C level, the higher your risk for diabetes and diabetic complications. A higher level also indicates poor blood sugar control.

The results of the A1C test are reported as a percentage, and the normal range for someone without diabetes is 4 to 5.6 percent. A1C levels of 5.7 to 6.4 percent indicate increased risk for diabetes or that someone already has prediabetes. For someone with diabetes, the American Diabetes Association recommends a goal of keeping A1C levels at less than 7 percent for adults. Levels at or near 8 percent indicate poor blood sugar control. People with type 2 diabetes should have the A1C test done every three months until it is determined that blood sugar levels are under control. Once sugar levels are under good control it will be up to your doctor to determine how often you should receive this test. In general it is recommended twice per year. It is important to note that people with conditions affecting hemoglobin, such as anemia, may get abnormal test results. In addition, taking supplements such as vitamin C and E can also affect test results, as can other health conditions such as high blood cholesterol levels, kidney disease, and liver disease.

Are there complications of type 2 diabetes that I need to worry about?

Type 2 diabetes is nothing to take lightly. There are plenty of serious health complications related to type 2 diabetes, especially if blood sugars are not properly managed. Some of these complications are:

> **Retinopathy:** *Retinopathy* is the term used to describe damage to the blood vessels of the retina in the eye. Prolonged periods of high blood sugar can damage the tiny blood vessels of the retina. This can cause the retina to become detached from the back of the eye,

causing double or blurry vision, seeing floaters, or experiencing dark spots over part of your vision. Detached retinas need immediate medical attention. Retinopathy is not always noticeable in the early stages and can develop for years without symptoms. It is not only important to control blood sugar but also blood pressure and cholesterol levels to help prevent this type of damage to your eyes. If you notice any changes in your vision, contact your eye doctor immediately. Diabetes can also increase the risk for other eye conditions such as glaucoma and cataracts.

Your Nutrition Solution Tidbit: Your doctor may report your A1C levels as eAG, or "average glucose," which still directly correlates to your A1C number. Your eAG may just be easier to understand because instead of being reported as a percentage, as in A1C, it is shown in the same units as you would normally see with your blood sugar levels (mg/dL).

☙ **Nephropathy, or Kidney Disease:** The longer you have diabetes, the higher your risk is for kidney disease, especially if blood sugar is not managed properly. The kidneys contain millions of tiny blood vessels that filter hazardous toxins from your blood. High blood sugar levels make the kidneys filter too much blood, and in time this begins to wear out the delicate filters of the kidneys and they begin to work less effectively. The damage to the kidneys is usually progressive, and if you have high blood pressure as well as type 2 diabetes the progress will be even quicker. If not addressed this can eventually lead to kidney failure. Keeping your blood sugar in check along with blood pressure is your first step to decreasing your risk for kidney disease. In addition, have your urine checked for protein once a year, keep your weight in a healthy range, do not smoke, limit your alcohol intake, exercise regularly, and eat a healthy diet to decrease your risk even further.

ℵ **Neuropathy:** Neuropathy is a disorder of the nerves. Having diabetes for many years along with prolonged high blood sugar levels can lead to nerve damage by injuring the blood vessels (capillaries) that nourish your nerves, especially in the legs. Symptoms can include tingling, numbness, or a burning pain that can begin at the tips of the toes and travel upward. Continued poorly controlled blood sugar can eventually cause a loss of feeling in affected limbs. Nerve damage in the feet and/or poor blood flow to the feet can also increase the risk of various foot complications. Neuropathy can also affect nerves in the digestive tract, causing nausea, vomiting, diarrhea, and/or constipation.

ℵ **Heart Disease:** Diabetes can dramatically increase your risk of heart disease and various cardiovascular issues such as coronary artery disease, heart attack, stroke, atherosclerosis (narrowing of the arteries), and high blood pressure. In fact, according to the American Heart Association, the risk for stroke is two to four times higher in people with diabetes, and the death rate after a heart attack is three times higher in diabetics with elevated fasting blood sugar levels.

Other complications from diabetes, especially in those with uncontrolled blood sugar levels, include hearing loss, lower-limb amputations, skin and mouth conditions, infections, osteoporosis, and Alzheimer's disease. Diabetes continues to be the primary cause of death for more than 71,000 Americans each year. So the answer to this questions is yes, there are serious complications related to type 2 diabetes—and plenty of them. The key to lowering your risk for almost all of these complications is to control your blood sugar, eat healthily, exercise, and simply take good care of yourself!

What does metabolic syndrome have to do with type 2 diabetes?

Metabolic syndrome is the term given for a group of risk factors that can greatly increase your risk for cardiovascular disease, stroke, and type 2 diabetes. In fact, studies have found that metabolic syndrome can be a strong predictor for type 2 diabetes.[1] You can have any of the risk factors for metabolic syndrome independently, such as high blood pressure, but when a person has other risk factors such as high cholesterol, abdominal obesity, and/or high fasting blood sugar, then she is diagnosed with metabolic syndrome and her condition becomes serious. This condition affects about 35 percent of all American adults. To be diagnosed with metabolic syndrome you must have at least three of the metabolic risk factors, which include:

- Excess abdominal obesity, or having an apple shape. Having a large waistline (40 inches or more for men and 35 inches or more for women) increases your risk for heart disease more than having excess fat in other parts of the body, such as the hips.

- A high blood triglyceride level (150 mg/dL or more) or being on medication to treat high triglycerides. Triglycerides are basically a type of fat that is found in your blood.

- A low HDL ("good" cholesterol) level of 40 mg/dL or less for men and 50 mg/dL or less for women, or being on medication to treat low HDL cholesterol. HDL cholesterol is "good" cholesterol because it helps to remove cholesterol from the arteries. If your HDL levels are low it puts you at a higher risk for heart disease.

- High blood pressure with a systolic (top number) of 130 mm Hg or greater and/or a diastolic (bottom number) of 85 mm Hg (millimeters of mercury) or greater, or being on medication to treat high blood pressure. Blood pressure is the force of blood that pushes against the walls of the arteries when your heart pumps blood. If the pressure is high and stays that way, in time it can begin to damage the heart and lead to problematic plaque buildup.

- High fasting blood sugar of 100 mg/dL or more, or being on medication to treat high blood sugar. Mild to moderate high blood sugar is usually a sign of prediabetes, which can be an early sign of type 2 diabetes.

- Insulin resistance or glucose intolerance such that your body cannot properly use insulin or blood sugar.

The major goal of treating metabolic syndrome is to decrease the risk for a heart attack. Treatment includes taking measures to lower LDL cholesterol, increase HDL cholesterol, lower blood pressure, and manage blood sugar. If type 2 diabetes has not yet developed, the next goal would be to take steps to prevent the onset. The main focus of treating metabolic syndrome is to manage the risk factors that are within your control, such as being overweight or obese, eating an unhealthy diet, and living an inactive lifestyle.

Your Nutrition Solution Tidbit: According to the National Diabetes Federation, people with metabolic syndrome are three times as likely to have a heart attack or stroke and twice as likely to die from it as people who do not have metabolic syndrome. People with metabolic syndrome have a five-fold greater risk of developing type 2 diabetes.

Who is most at risk for type 2 diabetes?

We have already discussed a few possible causes or risk factors for type 2 diabetes, including overweight/obesity, metabolic syndrome, insulin resistance, and prediabetes. Although not everyone with type 2 diabetes is overweight or obese, 85.2 percent are. In addition, type 2 diabetes has a strong genetic link and tends to run in families. If you have any of the risk factors for type 2 diabetes, you are encouraged to speak with your doctor about being screened for diabetes. The sooner you are diagnosed, the sooner you can begin to take steps to treat your condition and lower your risk for any serious health issues related to diabetes.

Other factors that put people at a higher risk for developing type 2 diabetes (many of them similar to those for prediabetes) include:

- A family history of type 2 diabetes; risk increases if a parent or sibling has it
- High blood pressure
- High blood cholesterol levels
- Having gestational diabetes during a pregnancy and/or giving birth to a baby weighing more than 9 pounds
- Consuming an unhealthy diet that includes too many of the unhealthy fats, too many simple carbohydrates, and not enough fiber on a regular basis

- Excessive alcohol intake
- A consistently sedentary lifestyle
- Being overweight or obese
- Carrying extra body fat in the abdominal area versus elsewhere, such as hips and thighs
- Ethnicity: certain groups of people have a higher risk of developing type 2 diabetes, including African Americans, Native Americans, Hispanic Americans, and Japanese Americans
- Increasing age: the risk for type 2 diabetes significantly rises after about age 45 and the risk rises even more after 65 years of age

Many of these factors, such as age and ethnicity, are out of your control, but the good news is that there are plenty of risk factors that you *are* able to change.

Can type 2 diabetes be reversed or cured?

Yes and no. Most people cannot turn back the clock to a point when they never had the disease, but it is possible to get to a point where you are managing your type 2 diabetes with a healthier diet and lifestyle and not relying on medication and/ or insulin. However, it is important to understand that living a healthier lifestyle is a treatment and must be followed for a lifetime to prevent type 2 diabetes symptoms from reoccurring. Much of whether you can actually reverse type 2 diabetes depends on how long you have had it, how severe it is, and whether you have inherited genes for the disease. In any case, exercise and a healthy diet are key steps to more easily managing type 2 diabetes.

Your Nutrition Solution Tidbit: Prediabetes is much more easily "reversed" than type 2 diabetes. If you have been diagnosed with prediabetes, taking steps now to reverse it can prevent you from eventually ending up with type 2 diabetes.

What are the signs and symptoms of type 2 diabetes?

Early detection of type 2 diabetes is the key to lowering your risk for serious health complications due to the disease. The sooner you are able to recognize the signs or symptoms, the sooner you can see your doctor to be properly diagnosed and begin treatment.

Common symptoms of type 2 diabetes include:

- Extreme thirst
- Feeling very hungry, especially after you have already eaten
- Frequent urination
- Dry mouth
- Extreme fatigue
- Blurry vision
- Tingling, pain, or numbness in the hands or feet
- Slow healing of cuts and bruises
- Unexplained headaches

Contact your doctor if you have experienced these types of symptoms and have not yet been diagnosed with type 2 diabetes. It is vitally important to be tested and start treatment as early as possible to lower your risk for serious health problems down the road. Sometimes symptoms can be so subtle that about a third of all people with type 2 diabetes don't even know they have it. Most often, symptoms gradually develop and worsen over time. Don't wait for your symptoms to get worse. If you have any risk factors and/or signs of diabetes, don't be afraid to ask your doctor to be tested.

How is type 2 diabetes diagnosed?

So you have risk factors and feel you may have a few of the symptoms just listed. Now what? What will your doctor do to see if you actually have type 2 diabetes? Testing will be done via a blood test and will include some of the tests we discussed previously, including fasting blood sugar (not eating or drinking anything but water for 8 hours), a 2-hour oral glucose tolerance test (OGTT), a random blood sugar test, and a hemoglobin A1C test. Once testing has been done, results must meet one of the following criteria for you to be diagnosed with type 2 diabetes. You must have:

- Some symptoms of diabetes and a random blood sugar level equal or greater to 200 mg/dL
- A fasting blood sugar level, on two separate tests, that is equal to or greater than 126 mg/dL
- A 2-hour OGTT test result that is equal to or greater than 200 mg/dL
- A hemoglobin A1C result that is 6.5 percent or higher

Before your diagnosis of diabetes is confirmed, your doctor will most likely repeat the same blood sugar test or do a different type of blood sugar test on another day.

What types of healthcare professionals will I need to see?

Your primary care physician will most likely diagnose your type 2 diabetes and then refer you to an endocrinologist, which is a doctor who specializes in hormonal disorders. This will be the doctor who will treat and help you manage your diabetes for the long term. Other healthcare professionals on your team may also include a registered dietitian nutritionist (RDN), a certified diabetes educator (CDE), a podiatrist (foot doctor), and an ophthalmologist (eye doctor).

> **Your Nutrition Solution Tidbit:** A certified Diabetes Educator (CDE) is a health professional, such as a dietitian, nurse, or pharmacist who possesses comprehensive knowledge and experience in the prevention, management, and education of diabetes as well as prediabetes. To become certified they must meet eligibility requirements and pass a certification exam.

What are my options for treatment? Will I need to take medication?

Once your diagnosis of type 2 diabetes is confirmed the next line of business will concern treatment options. Current recommendations by the American Diabetes Association state that individuals who have prediabetes or diabetes should receive individualized nutrition therapy provided by a registered dietitian nutritionist (RDN) who is familiar with the components of diabetes medical nutrition therapy (MNT). The first priority in treatment of type 2 diabetes is to educate and encourage individuals to implement lifestyle changes that will improve blood sugar levels, blood pressure, and dyslipidemia (high LDL, or "bad" cholesterol, high triglyceride levels, and low HDL, or "good" cholesterol). These lifestyle changes can include:

- Eating a healthier diet using many of the same nutrition recommendations that are used for the general public
- Losing weight if overweight or obese
- Monitoring blood sugar levels regularly
- Becoming physically active
- Taking diabetes medication or insulin therapy
- Taking medications to lower blood pressure and cholesterol

Some people with type 2 diabetes can manage their blood sugar by balancing a healthy diet, a healthy weight, and exercise, whereas others may need oral diabetes medication and/or insulin therapy in addition to those treatments. This decision will be made by you and your healthcare specialist and will depend on many factors, including your blood sugar levels and other health issues you may have.

Diabetes Medications

Different types of oral diabetes medications work in different ways to control blood sugar. Your doctor may use a combination of drugs from different classes to better control your blood sugar levels. As with most medications, there are possible side effects so you will have to weigh the pros and cons with your doctor to choose the best combination for you.

There are several classes of these oral medications available on the market today. As research continues look for these medications to change.

- **Sulfonylureas** stimulate the beta cells in your pancreas to produce and release more insulin in order to lower blood sugar. Examples include Glucotrol, Diabeta, Micronase, Glynase, and Amaryl. These medications have the same effect on blood glucose but differ in the possible side effects. Possible side effects include low blood sugar, upset stomach, and weight gain. These types of drugs are generally taken once or twice a day before meals.

- **Biguanides** help to improve your body's sensitivity to insulin and lower the production of glucose by the liver. Examples include Glucophage (metformin) and Riomet (liquid metformin). Possible side effects include gastrointestinal issues that usually go away after you have been on the medication for a while and also subside if the medication is taken with food. These types of drugs are usually taken twice daily.

- **Alpha-Glucosidase Inhibitors** help lower blood sugar levels by blocking the breakdown of starchy foods such as bread, potatoes, rice, and pasta in the intestines. Their action slows down the rise in blood sugar after consuming a meal. Examples include Glyset and Precose. Possible side effects include gastrointestinal issues that usually go away after you have been on the medication for a while. These drugs should be taken with the first bite of your meal.

- **Thiazolidinediones** make your body more sensitive to insulin, helping the insulin to work better in the muscle and fat. They also reduce glucose production in the liver. Examples include ACTOS and Avandia. Possible side effects include anemia, increased bone fractures in women, and complications with birth control medication. This medication should not be taken by anyone with congestive heart failure as it can cause or make this condition worse. People on these drugs are closely monitored for liver problems as well.

❧ **Meglitinides** stimulate the beta cells of the pancreas to produce more insulin. Examples include Starlix and Prandin. Possible side effects include low blood sugar, weight gain, upset stomach, back pain, and headache. These drugs are generally taken before each of your three daily meals.

❧ **DPP-4 Inhibitors** work by preventing the breakdown of GLP-1, which is a naturally occurring compound in the body that helps reduce blood glucose. GLP-1 is broken down very quickly, so by interfering with the breakdown of GLP-1, DPP-4 inhibitors allow it to remain active in the body longer, thereby lowering blood sugar levels only when they are elevated, including after meals. These drugs are able to improve A1C levels without causing hypoglycemia (low blood sugar). Examples include Januvia, Onglyza, Tradjenta, and Nesina. Possible side effects include runny nose, sore throat, and headache. These drugs do not tend to cause weight gain and have a neutral to positive effect on blood cholesterol levels.

❧ **SGLT2 (Sodium-Glucose Transporters) Inhibitors** work in the kidneys to cause excess glucose to be eliminated in the urine instead of reabsorbed and eventually released into the bloodstream. Examples include Invokana and Farxiga. These medications are fairly new. Because these medications increase the level of glucose in the urine, side effects can include yeast infections and urinary tract infections.

⩔ **Bile Acid Sequestrants (BAS)** are actually cholesterol-lowering medications that also tend to reduce blood sugar levels in people with diabetes. It is known how these medications reduces cholesterol levels (mainly LDL), but it is less known how they actually lower blood sugar levels. These medications are not absorbed into the bloodstream and therefore are often used for people with liver problems. Side effects can include gas and constipation.

⩔ **Oral Combination Therapy** is often used for better control of blood sugar levels. Because different medications all work in a different way to lower blood glucose levels, they are often used in combination with each other when a single medication does not have the desired effect.

Insulin Therapy

Some people with diabetes may need insulin therapy in addition to oral medication. This will depend on factors such as how well oral medications alone work for you, how long you have had diabetes, how high your blood sugar levels are, and your overall health. Insulin cannot be taken as an oral medication because it is broken down during digestion just like the protein in food is. Therefore insulin has to be injected into the fat under your skin in order for it to get into the bloodstream and be effective. Insulin can be injected with a device such as a fine needle and syringe or an insulin pen injector, which is most popular. There are many different types of insulin, in fact 20 different types sold in the United States currently. They differ in how quickly they work, when they peak, and how long they last. They include *rapid-acting insulin* such as Humalog and NovoLog; *regular or short-acting insulin* such as Humulin R and Novolin R; *intermediate-acting insulin* such as Humulin N and Novolin N; and *long-acting insulin* such as Levemir and Lantus. Depending on your individual needs, your doctor may prescribe a mixture of different types of insulin to use at different times of the day. Insulin is also available in different strengths, with U-100 being the most common. In the United States all insulin is manufactured in a laboratory.

> **Your Nutrition Solution Tidbit:** When taking either oral medications or insulin injections for control of blood sugars in type 2 diabetes, timing is everything. Your meals need to be spaced according to the medication and/or insulin you are taking and its period of peak action. In addition, the healthier your diet, the more effective medications and insulin will be. Taking either of these is not a green light to eat whatever you want! Your dietitian and/or certified diabetes educator will help you in timing and modifying your meals accordingly.

chapter 2

the nutrition connection and beyond

Now that you have a better understanding of exactly what type 2 diabetes is, we can take a deeper look into how nutrition can be the solution to managing this disease. This chapter will discuss nutrients, including carbohydrates, fat, protein, fiber, sodium, and cholesterol, and even some vitamins and minerals, and what role they play in managing type 2 diabetes. This chapter will help you to realize just how important your nutritional intake is to managing your disease for a lifetime.

The Macronutrients

Macronutrients are the main food components of our diet that provide calories, or fuel, for our body. These include carbohydrates, proteins, and fats. Each one of these macronutrients plays an important role in managing your blood sugar. How a particular food affects your blood sugar has to do in part with the combination of these macronutrients as well as the portion size you consume. There have been all types of "optimal mixes" of macronutrients suggested for diabetic diets, but the truth is there really isn't one combination of macronutrients that works best for *all* people with diabetes. According to the American Diabetes Association, the best mix of carbohydrates, proteins, and fats is one that correlates with each individual's circumstances. The best advice is to follow a diet that is recommended for all healthy adults and adjust from there according to your individual needs with the help of a registered dietitian nutritionist (RDN) and/or a certified diabetes educator (CDE). (We will talk more about healthy diets in Chapter 3.)

Carbohydrates

Carbohydrates, or "carbs," as they are more commonly known, provide fuel for our body in the form of glucose. They are found in fruits, vegetables (especially starchy vegetables), dairy products, breads, cereals, rices, and pastas. Unlike proteins and fats, the amount of carbs you consume directly influences your blood sugar levels because carbs are broken down directly into sugar very early in the digestion process. This makes carbs a significant element in the diet of people with type 2 diabetes. There are three main types of carbohydrates in food:

1. **Starches** (also called complex carbohydrates) include some vegetables, such as peas, corn, and potatoes;

dried beans and lentils; and grains (both refined and whole grains), such as breads, pasta, rice, oats, and barley. Starches are single sugars that are bonded together.

2. **Sugars** (also called simple carbohydrates) come in two main categories: (1) naturally occurring, such as the sugar found in fruits, milk, and other dairy products, and (2) added sugars, such as those added during processing of foods like cookies, pastries, some cereals, and the list goes on and on. Simple sugars, such as table sugar, honey, cane sugar, molasses, syrup, high-fructose corn syrup, powdered sugar, beet sugar, and brown sugar. Sometimes you will find sugar listed by its chemical name, sucrose or fructose. You can recognize other chemical names for sugar as they all end in "-ose."

3. **Fiber**, also considered a carbohydrate, comes strictly from plant foods and is the indigestible part of these foods. Good sources of fiber include whole-grain foods, fruits, vegetables, beans, and nuts.

Your Nutrition Solution Tidbit: Although low-carbohydrate diets might seem to be a logical approach to lowering your blood sugar, it is much the opposite. Foods that contain carbohydrates are an important source of energy, fiber, vitamins, and minerals, and they are a necessary component in the diets of people with diabetes. Keep in mind that too low of a blood sugar level can be just as dangerous as too high of a blood sugar level. It is about balancing your carbs, not cutting them out.

Monitoring your carbohydrate intake, whether by using a carb-counting method, the healthy plate method (discussed later), or experience-based estimation, is part of a key strategy in achieving glycemic control. The amount of carbs you consume will directly impact your blood sugar, so keeping track of them is a must. (We will discuss carb counting and the healthy plate method in Chapter 3.)

The recommendation for carbohydrates in diabetes management by the American Diabetes Association is a dietary pattern that includes carbs from fruits, vegetables, whole grains, legumes, and low-fat milk. Although there is no true recommended percentage of daily carbohydrates for diabetes, most experts recommend a general intake of about 45 to 60 grams of carbohydrates at each meal. That amount may vary if you are taking oral medications and/or insulin injections.

When you do eat carbs, make them count! In other words, because you are going to have to moderate your carbohydrate intake, make sure the carbs you do include in your diet plan are going to provide you with the most bang for your buck, or the most nutritional value for the calories.

Whole Grains versus Refined Grains

Always strive to choose whole grains instead of refined grains. Whole grains include the entire grain kernel—bran, germ, and endosperm. These include foods such as oatmeal, brown rice, wild rice, popcorn, whole-wheat flour, quinoa, bran, and whole-grain pasta. Whole grains are full of nutritional value and fiber to help slow down the absorption of sugar into the bloodstream. Refined grains, on the other hand, have been milled, which is a process that removes the bran and germ from the grain. This process removes essential nutrients and fiber as well. These foods include white flour, white rice, white breads, sugary cereals, and white pastas. Many refined grains are enriched, meaning some of the nutrients lost after milling are added back in. However, fiber is not one of them, so refined grains have a much lower fiber content and a higher glycemic index, and they will raise blood sugar much faster. When choosing whole-grain foods look for the word "whole" on the label or in the ingredients. If, for example, the label states "wheat bread," it is not a whole grain; if it states "whole wheat bread," then it is. Check out *http://wholegrainscouncil.org* for more info on whole grains.

The Glycemic Index

The glycemic index (GI) measures how much each gram of available carbohydrate (total carbohydrate minus the fiber) in a single food affects your blood sugar level. The glycemic index only pertains to foods that contain carbohydrates, so proteins and fats do not have a GI. Foods are ranked with an "index" by how they compare to pure glucose, which has a GI of 100 per 50 grams. A food with a high GI raises blood sugar higher and faster, whereas a food with a medium or low GI does the opposite. This index can sometimes be helpful, but the problem is that the GI deals with one food at a time, and eating foods in combination with each other (as most of us do every day!) can change the way each food affects blood sugar. So, if you are eating the food alone the GI may be a good tool to use, but if you are eating several different foods together in a meal it may not work as well. The key in that case would be to balance a high-GI food with low-GI foods in the same meal to create a balance. Foods that tend to have a lower GI are those that contain fiber and fat. Both of these nutrients slow down the absorption of glucose into the blood stream. Other factors can also affect the GI, such as the ripeness of a fruit, or the processing or cooking method. The problem to consider when thinking about the GI and managing blood glucose is that the glycemic index represents the *type* of carbohydrate in a food and not the *amount* of that carbohydrate. Because the amount of carbs you eat is also essential in controlling blood sugar, you should not use the GI as your sole method for controlling your blood sugar. Another issue is that some very nutritious foods have a higher GI than some not-so-nutritious foods. It is important to remember that whether a food has a high or low glycemic index does not necessarily equate to whether a food is healthy or not.

Here are some examples of low-GI foods (55 or less):

- 100-percent stone-ground whole-wheat bread
- Pumpernickel bread
- Corn/wheat tortilla
- Brown rice
- Oatmeal or oat bran
- Legumes and lentils
- Avocados
- Apples
- Hummus
- Nuts
- Milk

Here are some examples of medium-GI foods (56–69):

- Sweet potatoes
- Couscous
- Bananas
- Grapes

- White spaghetti noodles
- White rice

Here are some examples of high-GI foods (70 or more):
- White breads
- Baked goods
- Crackers
- White potatoes
- Kiwis
- Pineapples
- Watermelon

Glycemic Load

The glycemic load is based on the glycemic index but takes into account not only the effect on blood sugar but also the amount of carbohydrates in the food. A food's glycemic load is calculated by multiplying a food's glycemic index by the amount of carbohydrates it contains. Because the glycemic load includes both components, a specific food can have a high glycemic index but a low glycemic load, making it a better choice than it may have originally appeared to be. Using glycemic load can help to control blood sugar levels, but as with the GI it should be used along with other methods because meal planning includes all food groups, not only foods that contain carbs.

Some examples of foods with a low glycemic load (10 and under) are:
- High-fiber fruits and vegetables (excluding white potatoes)

- Bran cereals
- Most dried beans, legumes, and lentils
- Most nuts
- Milk

Some examples of foods with a medium glycemic load (11–19) are:

- Brown rice
- Oatmeal
- Whole-grain bread
- Bulgur
- Whole-grain pasta
- Sweet potatoes

Some examples of foods with a high glycemic load (20+) are:

- White potatoes
- French fries
- Couscous
- Refined (sugary) breakfast cereals
- White breads
- White pastas

Your Nutrition Solution Tidbit: The American Diabetes Association states that using the glycemic index and glycemic load may provide a modest additional benefit compared to when total carbohydrate intake is considered alone. Both GI and GL can be confusing tools so it is best to seek the help of a RDN and/or CDE if using this as a method to control blood sugar.

Proteins

Protein foods include mostly meats, poultry, eggs, and fish, but there are also non-animal protein sources, such as beans, lentils, and soy foods that contain not only protein but also carbohydrates. The biggest difference is that meat and most other animal sources do not affect blood sugar, whereas non-animal sources do because they contain carbohydrates. However, that doesn't mean that you should consume a high-protein diet made up of only animal protein sources to help control blood sugar. High-protein diets can be taxing on the kidneys and add high saturated fat content (contributing to heart disease and stroke) to your diet, depending on the types of protein sources you choose. According to the Dietary Reference Intakes (*http:// fnic.nal.usda.gov/dietary-guidance/dietary-reference-intakes*), for a healthy individual an acceptable macronutrient distribution for protein is about 10 to 35 percent of total calorie intake. The recommended daily allowance (RDA) is 0.8 grams of high-quality protein per kilogram of body weight per day.

High-quality protein sources are those that provide all nine of the essential amino acids (the building blocks of protein), and include meat, poultry, fish/seafood, eggs, milk, cheese, and soy (the only plant-based protein source that is considered a high-quality protein). Protein sources that are not considered high quality because they do not contain all nine essential amino acids are usually plant protein sources such as grains, cereals, nuts, beans, and vegetables. But just because a food does not contain high-quality protein, that does not mean the food is not healthy; it just means that it doesn't contribute to protein as well as high-quality proteins do. However, these other protein foods are usually lower in saturated fat and cholesterol and are good sources of dietary fiber. If you are vegetarian and consuming only plant-based protein sources, your protein intake should be greater than the 0.8 grams per kilogram to account for the mixed protein quality in foods. The recommended dietary intake of protein for people with type 2 diabetes is very similar to that for the general public, and, according to the American Diabetes Association, should not exceed 20 percent of total calorie intake. When choosing animal-based protein sources your best choices include skinless chicken and turkey, lean pork fish (especially salmon), and select grades of extra lean/lean beef that has been trimmed of visible fat. Keep in mind that when you choose plant-based protein choices, they need to be added into your carbohydrate calculations. In addition, even though soy-based foods make a good protein choice, they are more processed and therefore tend to have a higher glycemic index.

Your Nutrition Solution Tidbit: Although fish is a healthy protein option, certain types of fish contain mercury—some more than others. For most of us this is not an issue, but for women who may become pregnant, pregnant women, nursing mothers, and young children it can be a health concern. For this reason the FDA and the EPA (Environmental Protection Agency) issued an advisory to these people to avoid some types of fish that are higher in mercury. The advisory warns for this specific population to not eat shark, swordfish, king mackerel, or tilefish because they contain higher levels of mercury. They can eat up to 12 ounces a week (two average meals) of a variety of fish and shellfish that are lower in mercury. Five of the most commonly eaten fish, low in mercury, are shrimp, canned light tuna, salmon, pollock, and catfish. Albacore (white) tuna has more mercury then canned light tuna, so this population may eat up to 6 ounces of albacore tuna per week. Check local advisories about the safety of fish caught locally. If you cannot find advice, eat up to 6 ounces per week of fish caught from local waters and do not consume any other fish that week. These same recommendations hold true for young children, but they are to be served smaller portions.

Fats

Because diabetes can increase your risk of heart disease it is important to eat foods that are lower in fat, especially saturated and trans fat, to keep your risk as low as possible. Both of these fats contribute greatly to heart disease and other health complications. In addition, limiting fat can also lower calorie intake, making it easier to lose excess weight that may also be aggravating your type 2 diabetes. Research has shown that people with type 2 diabetes who balance protein and fat along with their carbohydrates are able to control their blood sugars better, because fats help lower the blood-sugar response to other foods it is consumed with. However, balancing is key. Meals with too much fat, especially the unhealthy fats, can have the opposite effect. The solution is not getting too much fat, and choosing the right ones.

Not all fats are created equal. There are different types of fat, some healthy and some not so healthy. Fats *do* matter in our diet. They are necessary and an essential nutrient, as we could not survive without them. However, fats (both healthy and unhealthy) are twice as high in calories as carbohydrates and protein, so be mindful about your portion sizes when it comes to fat sources. A little bit goes a long way!

Monounsaturated Fats

These are "healthy" fats and a good source of vitamin E, which is an antioxidant that most of us need more of in our diets. According to the American Heart Association, monounsaturated fats, when used to replace saturated and/or trans fats, can help to lower total cholesterol and LDL ("bad") blood cholesterol, reducing the risk for heart disease and stroke. Besides lowering cholesterol, the vitamin E that most of these foods contain is a powerful antioxidant that has been associated with reducing the risk for heart disease. Research has shown that olive oil, which is high in monounsaturated fats, can reduce inflammation and possibly protect from some forms of cancer.[1] In addition, they can help to increase insulin sensitivity, helping the body to better utilize glucose. Foods highest in monounsaturated fatty acids include:

- Olive oil and olives
- Canola and peanut oil
- Sunflower and sesame oil
- Avocados
- Nuts, including hazelnuts, macadamia nuts, almonds, Brazil nuts, cashews, and pecans
- Seeds, including sesame seeds and pumpkin seeds
- Peanut butter

Polyunsaturated Fats

These are another "healthy" fat. When polyunsaturated fats are consumed in moderation and used to replace saturated fats and/or trans fats in the diet they can help reduce total cholesterol, lower LDL ("bad") blood cholesterol levels, and lower blood triglyceride levels, thus lowering the risk for heart disease and stroke. These types of unsaturated fats include omega-6 and omega-3 fatty acids, which are essential to add to our diet because the body cannot produce them. Polyunsaturated fats have many of the same health benefits as monounsaturated fats. Foods highest in polyunsaturated fatty acids include:

- Vegetable oils such as soybean, corn, and safflower Oils
- Nuts, including walnuts, pine nuts, and butternuts
- Seeds, including sunflower seeds, flaxseeds, and sesame seeds
- Fatty fish and seafood (in the form of omega-3 fatty acids)

Omega-3 fatty acids are a group of polyunsaturated fatty acids. They stand on their own as a healthy fat because of the myriad of health benefits they provide. These fats play a crucial role in brain function as well as normal growth and development of the body. Omega-3 fatty acids are proven to help to reduce inflammation and may have the power to reduce the risk for heart disease, cancer, and arthritis. They may help lower total cholesterol, increase HDL ("good") cholesterol, lower triglycerides, lower blood pressure, possibly help alleviate some of the symptoms of depression and other psychological disorders, improve skin disorders, and the list goes on as more research is completed. Both the American Diabetes Association and the American Heart Association advocate eating fatty fish as a safe and effective way to obtain the heart-healthy benefits of omega-3 fatty acids.

Omega-3 fatty acids are found mostly in fatty fish in the form of EPA (eicosapentaeonic) and DHA (docoshexaeonic). These two types of omega-3 fatty acids are potent forms and provide the greatest health potential. Omega-3 fatty acids can also be found in a variety of plant foods such as walnuts, soybeans, flaxseeds, pumpkin seeds, and numerous nut oils in the form of ALA (alpha linolenic acid), which is a precursor for EPA and DHA. However, ALA is not quite as potent and doesn't have the same amount of benefits as the fat found in fish.

Just two servings a week of foods high in omega-3 fatty acids can give you what you need to reap their health benefits, but as with the other healthy fats, they need to *replace* the unhealthy fats, rather than merely being an addition to your diet. And don't go overboard. Too much omega-3, especially in the form of supplements, can have negative health implications for some people. Speak with your doctor before starting an omega-3 or fish oil supplement. Foods highest in omega-3 fatty acids are:

- Salmon
- Mackerel
- Halibut
- Tuna
- Herring

Your Nutrition Solution Tidbit: Some foods on the market today, including eggs, yogurt, peanut butter, bread, and pasta, are fortified with omega-3 fatty acids (usually in the form of ALA). These fortified foods usually contain very little of this healthy fatty acid, and you would need to eat a lot of the food to get close to what is recommended. The additional omega-3 fatty acids found in these foods aren't harmful, but you shouldn't substitute these "functional foods" for ones that naturally contain omega-3 fatty acids.

Saturated Fats

Saturated fats are most definitely one of the bad guys in the fat group. They are one of the main causes of high blood cholesterol levels, even more so than dietary cholesterol itself. Because many of these foods are *also* high in cholesterol, it's a double whammy! Saturated fat triggers the liver to make more cholesterol—the LDL, or "bad," cholesterol. This all adds up to a higher risk for heart disease and stroke as well as some types of cancer. Saturated fats are found naturally in most animal-based foods such as meat, poultry, butter, and whole or reduced-fat milk and milk products. In addition, many baked goods as well and fried foods carry high levels of saturated fat. Even though most vegetable oils are a bigger source of unsaturated fat, there are a few that are more saturated, such as coconut oil, palm oil, and palm kernel oil. Foods highest in saturated fats include:

- High-fat meats
- Lard
- Butter
- Some baked goods
- High-fat or full-fat dairy products

Your Nutrition Solution Tidbit: Just a small reduction in saturated fat can go a long way. A report by the National Cholesterol Education Program recognized that a 1-percent decrease in dietary saturated fat led to a 2-percent decrease in LDL ("bad") cholesterol, which led to a 2-percent decrease in heart disease risk.

Trans Fats

One of the worst fats to add to your diet is trans fat. This type of fat is created when a liquid vegetable oil is made more solid by the addition of hydrogen through a process called *hydrogenation*. These more solid fats gained popularity with manufacturers because they increase the shelf life and flavor of many baked and processed foods. Trans fat has received more attention lately because researchers are finding out just how dangerous it can be to our health. Trans fats raise LDL (bad) cholesterol and lower your HDL (good) cholesterol. In fact, some experts believe they can raise LDL cholesterol even more than saturated fats can. Consuming these fats will increase your risk for heart disease and stroke, and they are also associated with a higher risk for developing type 2 diabetes. In January of 2006, the FDA required that all manufacturers begin adding trans fat amounts to their nutrition facts panel on food labels to make it easier for consumers to know just how much trans fat they are eating. With this change many manufacturers began taking trans fat out of their products. However, if the trans fat has been removed it has most likely been replaced with another type of fat, such as saturated fat, so check the nutrition facts panel. Most experts agree that the less trans fat you eat, the better. The American Heart Association recommends limiting the amount of trans fat you consume to less than 1 percent of your total daily calories. For example, if you need 2,000 calories per day that means you must get no more than 20 of those calories from trans fats, which is less than 2 grams a day. You can decrease the amount of trans fat you eat by including more fruits, vegetables, whole grains, and fat-free or low-fat dairy products to your diet, as well as leaner cuts of meat, poultry without the skin, fish and seafood, legumes, nuts, and seeds. Check labels for the amount of trans fat and scan ingredient lists for *hydrogenated* vegetable oils. Foods highest in trans fats include:

- Fried foods
- Commercial baked goods
- Some stick margarines
- Some fast foods such as French fries
- Some snack foods

> **Your Nutrition Solution Tidbit:** Even products that state "trans-fat free" can have up to 0.5 grams of trans fat per serving by labeling law definitions. This can add up quickly, especially if you are eating more than one serving. Even if the label states "trans-fat free," look on the ingredient list for "hydrogenated oil" or "partially hydrogenated oil" to see if the product really contains any trans fats.

Tips for Controlling Your Fat Intake

Because the intake of too many unhealthy fats and too few healthy fats can negatively affect your heart health, and because people with type 2 diabetes are already at an increased risk for heart disease, it is important to pay special attention to this nutrient. Here are a few tips to help you lower your total fat intake as well as increase healthy fats and decrease bad fats:

- Select lean cuts of meat, such as skinless poultry, pork, and lean red meats, and watch portion size. Choose fish, seafood, and plant-based proteins such as soy foods and legumes more often.
- When preparing foods stay away from frying and instead bake, broil, grill, roast, or boil.

ا Choose low-fat or fat-free dairy products and remember to include them in your daily carbohydrate counts.

ا Use low-fat vegetable-based cooking spray when preparing foods, and/or consider using cholesterol-lowering margarines that contain *stanols* or *sterols* in place of butter or stick margarine.

ا Use heart-healthy liquid vegetable oils that contain polyunsaturated or monounsaturated fats such as extra virgin olive oil or canola oil for cooking, dressings, and/or as a substitute for butter.

ا Create your own salad dressings instead of using commercial dressings, which can often be overly processed and full of saturated fats and sugar. Mix extra virgin olive oil, vinegar, and your favorite herbs and spices for a quick and healthier dressing.

ا When baking try replacing some of the fat with applesauce or other pureed fruit. Use light or extra-light olive oil for baking cakes or muffins.

ا Choose fat-free milk over whole or low-fat milk. Fat-free milk has as much calcium, vitamin D, and other essential nutrients as whole milk, but minus the saturated fat and calories.

ا Try using low-fat yogurt to replace sour cream in recipes or baking.

ا Replace one egg with two egg whites in recipes to cut back on fat and cholesterol.

Your Nutrition Solution Tidbit: Recommendations for dietary fat and cholesterol in diabetes management are as follows:

ا Limit saturated fat to less than 7 percent of total calories

- Minimize intake of trans fat
- In individuals with diabetes, limit dietary cholesterol to less than 200 mg per day
- Consume two or more servings of fish per week (with the exception of commercially fried fish filets) to provide n-3 polyunsaturated fatty acids.

The Micronutrients

Micronutrients are different from macronutrients because they are needed in only very small quantities. In addition, they do not provide energy in the form of calories and therefore do not directly affect blood sugar levels. Nevertheless, they are essential to our health and the proper functioning of our body. We know "micronutrients" better as vitamins and minerals. Problems with micronutrients occur when there is a deficiency. Currently there is no clear-cut evidence that additional vitamin and mineral supplementation is beneficial to those people with type 2 diabetes who do not have underlying deficiencies. That being said, because many of us don't get the daily micronutrients we need from diet alone, a general multivitamin/ mineral supplement is something to consider. It helps to ensure we are getting what we need daily. Always speak with your doctor before starting any type of supplementation. Eating a healthy, well-balanced diet daily with foods that provide all of these nutrients is your best bet.

Vitamin D

Vitamin D, a fat-soluble vitamin, has long been recognized as necessary for strong bones, and current research is beginning to reveal that the need for this vitamin goes much further in protecting our body from a host of health issues. Low blood levels of vitamin D are now being associated with an increased risk of death from cardiovascular disease, high blood pressure, cognitive impairment in older people, depression, some cancers, asthma in children, and the risk for insulin resistance and type 2 diabetes. Low vitamin D levels are often found among people with type 2 diabetes. Researchers are currently exploring whether vitamin D may have a direct impact on mood and blood pressure in those with type 2 diabetes.[2] Ongoing research is also discovering that vitamin D, along with calcium, may play a role in the secretion and action of insulin.

Our body produces vitamin D in response to sunlight, and we can also get it from food. However, it is difficult to get all we need from these two sources, and intake does not always guarantee absorption. In addition to sunlight, there are only a few food sources that naturally contain vitamin D, such as fatty fish and fish oils. A few others, such as beef liver, egg yolks, and cheese, contain only small amounts. Other foods that do not contain vitamin D naturally but are fortified with the vitamin include fortified milk, yogurt, breakfast cereals, and orange juice.

Some groups of people who are at higher risk for vitamin D deficiency are:

- People with type 2 diabetes
- Vegetarians who eat no animal foods
- People with dark skin and/or who do not get enough sunlight
- People who do not get sunlight all year long
- Older adults (with age, the kidneys have a harder time converting vitamin D to its active form, thus increasing the risk for deficiency)

- People with medical issues such as Crohn's or celiac disease that can inhibit the intestines from absorbing vitamin D from foods
- Obese people (fat cells can alter vitamin D's release into the blood)

Finding out if you have low vitamin D levels is as easy as a blood test. Although we should always start with food as the best way to supplement our diet, the small amounts of vitamin D found in food make it difficult. If you feel you are not getting enough vitamin D or you are at a higher risk for vitamin D deficiency (as determined by the previous list), speak with your doctor about being tested and possibly adding a supplement to your current diet. Taking a vitamin D supplement is generally safe, but taking too much and/or taking it with certain medications can cause side effects, so speak with your doctor first about the correct dosage for you.

Your Nutrition Solution Tidbit: The Recommended dietary allowance (RDA) for vitamin D is 600 IU (international units) for adults 18 years and older and 800 IU for those adults 71 years and older. These amounts are based on minimal sun exposure. The upper tolerable limit, or the amount that is likely safe when taking supplements, is 4,000 IU. If you need vitamin D supplementation your doctor will determine the correct dosage for your condition.

Magnesium

Magnesium is a mineral that is abundant in foods as well as in the body. It is also available as a dietary supplement, and it is added to many foods and medications, such as antacids. Just about every organ in the body, including the heart, muscles, and kidneys, needs magnesium in some way. This mineral also contributes to the makeup of our teeth and bones, and, even more important, it helps to regulate blood sugar levels, activates enzymes, contributes to energy production, and helps to regulate our body's levels of calcium, copper, zinc, potassium, vitamin D, and other nutrients.

Although magnesium is abundant in many foods, most people still do not get what they need due to poor dietary intake. Magnesium can be found mostly in whole grains, some nuts and seeds, legumes (especially black beans and soy beans), and green leafy vegetables, as well as tofu, wheat bran, whole-wheat flour, oat flour, bran cereals, oatmeal, and some herbs and spices. Although people don't always get all the magnesium they need through food, it is rare to be deficient in magnesium. However, certain medical conditions can upset the balance of magnesium levels—including diabetes. Excessive vomiting, diarrhea, and sweating; heavy menstrual periods for women; too much sodium, alcohol, caffeine, and soft drinks; and prolonged stress can also lower magnesium levels in the body. A deficiency of magnesium can manifest in muscle spasms, anxiety, restless leg syndrome, sleep problems, irritability, abnormal heart rhythms, low blood pressure, confusion, weakness, and even seizures. Research has found that getting enough magnesium can enhance the effectiveness of conventional treatment for conditions such as asthma, depression, fibromyalgia, arrhythmia and heart failure, high blood pressure, migraine headaches, osteoporosis, restless leg syndrome, premenstrual syndrome, and, last but not least, type 2 diabetes.[3]

People with type 2 diabetes are often found to be low in magnesium, which can make blood glucose control even tougher. Studies have found that getting more magnesium in the diet may help protect against developing type 2 diabetes. Taking magnesium supplements may help with blood sugar control and insulin sensitivity for some people with type 2 diabetes or prediabetes. If you are not able to get all of the magnesium you need through food and/or your doctor determines you need to increase this mineral, there are multiple forms of magnesium supplementation available. These include magnesium citrate, magnesium gluconate, and magnesium lactate. The body easily absorbs all of these forms. Other familiar sources include magnesium hydroxide, which is often found in laxatives and antacids, as well as magnesium sulfate, which is often used orally as a laxative or found in multivitamin supplements. Magnesium supplements can have potential side effects, some serious for people with heart and kidney disease, and can also interact with some medications as well. Too much magnesium through food doesn't seem to be a problem, but taking large quantities of magnesium through supplements or as a laxative can have serious health consequences. Always check with your doctor and continue under his or her supervision when taking a magnesium supplement. Your doctor may also recommend a B complex vitamin because the level of vitamin B6 in the body determines how much magnesium will be absorbed into the cells. Magnesium competes with calcium for absorption and can cause a calcium deficiency if your calcium levels are already on the low side.

Your Nutrition Solution Tidbit: The recommended dietary allowance (RDA) for magnesium for adult females ages 19 to 30 is 310 milligrams (mg) per day, and 320 mg for those females 31 years and

older. These levels increase slightly during pregnancy and breastfeeding. For adult males ages 19
to 30 the RDA is 400 mg per day, and 420 mg for
those males 31 years and older.. If you need magnesium supplementation your doctor will determine
the correct dosage for your condition.

Chromium

Chromium is a trace mineral that is essential for normal
glucose metabolism. Chromium is known to enhance the action of insulin. Deficiency has been found to lead to impaired
glucose tolerance. Though we don't need a lot of chromium,
it is widely distributed in our food supply. Most chromium-
containing foods, such as meat, whole-grain foods, milk and
milk products, some fruits and vegetables, and spices, provide
only small amounts. Although you may eat plenty of foods that
include chromium, very little is actually absorbed into the intestines; the rest is excreted from the body. Vitamin C and
the B vitamin niacin both help to enhance the absorption of
chromium.

An actual deficiency of chromium is rare. Research has
found that older adults may be more vulnerable to low levels
of chromium. At present more research is being done to determine whether supplementation with chromium may be helpful
in the treatment of impaired glucose tolerance and type 2 diabetes. Few serious effects from taking chromium supplementation have been noted, so the Food and Drug Administration
has not set a Tolerable Upper Intake Level (UL) at this point.
However, some medications can interact with chromium supplements, so always speak with your doctor before supplementing your diet with this trace mineral.

Your Nutrition Solution Tidbit: The Adequate Intake (AI) for chromium is 25 micrograms (mcg) per day for females ages 19 to 50 years, and 20 mcg for females ages 51 and older. The daily AI increases slightly during pregnancy and breastfeeding. For males ages 19 to 50 years the daily AI is 35 mcg, and 30 mcg for males ages 51 and older.

Antioxidants

Vitamin C and E, two powerful antioxidants, are of interest in the possible treatment of type 2 diabetes. Antioxidants neutralize or inactivate free radicals that can cause damage to the body in many ways, including cancer, heart disease, and nerve damage. Some experts believe that people with type 2 diabetes use up their stores of antioxidants like vitamins C and E faster, therefore increasing their requirements. As a result, some studies suggest that people with diabetes tend to have lower levels of vitamin C in their body.

Vitamin C is a water-soluble vitamin abundant in many fruits and vegetables, and is often added to cereals and other fortified foods. The body cannot store vitamin C, so serious side effects from too much vitamin C are rare. However, taking more than 2,000 mg daily is not recommended because doses that high can lead to stomach issues, diarrhea, and even kidney stones.

Vitamin E, a fat-soluble vitamin, may help prevent heart disease and plays an important role in preventing kidney and eye damage, all of which are common problems for people with type 2 diabetes. Good sources of vitamin E include vegetable oils, margarine, nuts, seeds, eggs, and leafy greens as well as fortified foods. Vitamin E supplements can be harmful to people who take blood thinners and certain other medications. Speak with your doctor before considering a vitamin C and/or vitamin E supplement.

Your Nutrition Solution Tidbit: The RDA for vitamin C for females 19 years of age and older is 75 mg per day with a slight increase during pregnancy and breastfeeding. For males who are 19 years of age and older the RDA for vitamin C is 90 mg per day. The upper tolerable limit for all adults is 2,000 mg per day.

The RDA for vitamin E for both males and females 19 years of age and older is 15 mg per day with a slight increase during breastfeeding for women. The upper tolerable intake level for all adults is 1,000 mg per day.

B Vitamins

People with type 2 diabetes tend to be deficient in the water-soluble vitamin B12. In addition, some oral diabetes medications, including metformin, increase the risk for B12 deficiency. This vitamin might also help lessen some of the complications associated with long-term type 2 diabetes. Vitamin B12 is essential for metabolism of homocysteine, an amino acid. When vitamin B12 is too low, blood levels of homocysteine rise. High levels of this amino acid have been associated with diabetic retinopathy, a complication that causes damage to the blood vessels of the eye. In addition, high homocysteine levels are also linked to cardiovascular disease, for which we know people with type 2 diabetes are already at higher risk. Vitamin B12 has shown some effectiveness in minimizing some symptoms associated with diabetic neuropathy, which is painful nerve damage that effects mostly the legs and feet. You can find B12 in a large variety of animal foods as well as some fortified foods.

Folic acid, another B vitamin, also tends to be lower in those with type 2 diabetes and is another vitamin that assists in lowering levels of homocysteine in the body. As with B12, taking metformin can increase the risk for a deficiency of folic acid. Folic acid can be found in foods such as dark green leafy vegetables, citrus fruits, fruit juices, beans, nuts, dairy products, and whole grains. In the United States, folic acid is added to most enriched grain products such as cereals, breads, flours, and pastas. Before supplementing with any B vitamin, speak with your doctor. It is never a good idea to take more than what is needed of any single vitamin or mineral.

Your Nutrition Solution Tidbit: The RDA for B12 is 2.4 mcg (micrograms) for both males and females 19 years of age and older. That rises during pregnancy and breastfeeding for women.

The RDA for folic acid is 400 mcg for both males and females 19 years of age and older. That also rises during pregnancy and breastfeeding for women.

Other Significant Nutrients

Fiber

High-fiber foods are very helpful for blood sugar control and management of type 2 diabetes. Foods high in fiber slows down digestion and promote the gradual release of insulin and a slower rise in blood pressure. Fiber is a type of complex carbohydrate that is found only in plants and is frequently referred to as "roughage." It is the indigestible part of plant foods. Unlike other carbohydrates, the body does not digest or absorb fiber entirely, so it contributes very few calories. Because of this, fiber is not truly considered a nutrient; however, you can still find it listed on food nutrient labels to help you choose fiber-rich foods.

There are two types of dietary fiber: soluble fiber and insoluble fiber. Both types of fiber benefit the body in many ways, from promoting regularity and preventing constipation to decreasing the risk for colon cancer as well as other types of cancers. In addition, fiber helps to lower LDL ("bad") cholesterol levels, reduce the risk for heart disease, and regulate blood sugar levels. As if that weren't enough, high-fiber foods can also help you to feel fuller longer after you eat, which in turn can keep you from nibbling when you shouldn't. And let's face it: fewer calories usually means weight loss! Although fiber isn't the magic cure for weight loss, if you replace some of those high-fat and high-sugar foods with foods that are healthy and higher in fiber, it most certainly can help. Even though fiber isn't truly considered a nutrient, it is still an important part of a healthy and well-balanced diet. Fiber can be found in loads of healthy foods, including fruits, vegetables, legumes/beans, oatmeal, whole grains, soy foods, lentils, nuts, and seeds. How much fiber you need daily depends on your gender and age. As long as you stick close to the recommended servings of fruits, vegetables, and whole grains and often throw in some legumes/beans, nuts, and seeds you should be able to meet your requirements.

Here are a few easy ways to increase your daily fiber and in turn help to control blood sugar levels:

- Start your day with a bowl of whole-grain cereal, either hot or cold, and top it with sliced fresh fruit.
- Make the switch from refined carbs to whole-grain breads, whole-wheat pastas, and brown or wild rice. You might even like the taste better!
- Add barley, beans, lentils, and split peas to salads, soups, casseroles, and stews.

- Grab a piece of fresh fruit when you get that afternoon sweet tooth.

- Do not overcook vegetables. Instead, lightly steam them to keep the fiber intact.

- Substitute part whole-wheat flour for white refined flour in baked goods.

- Sneak fiber into a sandwich by adding shredded carrots, sliced cucumbers, sliced tomato, raw spinach, and/or sprouts in between two slices of whole-wheat bread.

- Add nuts or low-fat granola to your favorite yogurt.

- Try dried fruits, which are higher in fiber than canned or fresh fruits.

- Leave the skin or peel on fruits and vegetables when possible, and wash them thoroughly before eating. Most of the fiber in fruits and vegetables is found in and around the skin.

- Read food labels and choose foods that are higher in fiber. Keep these nutritional claims in mind:

  - "Good Source of Fiber": 3 to less than 5 grams of fiber

  - "High in Fiber," "Rich in Fiber," "Excellent Source of Fiber": 5 grams of fiber or more (20 percent or more of your daily value)

Your Nutrition Solution Tidbit: The recommendations by the Institute of Medicine's Food and Nutrition Board state that adult women under 50 years of age need 25 grams of fiber daily, and women over 50 years of age need 21 grams daily. That amount increases during pregnancy and breastfeeding. Adult men under 50 years of age need 38 grams daily, and men over 50 years of age need 30 grams daily.

According to the American Diabetes Association, people with type 2 diabetes are encouraged to choose a variety of fiber-containing foods daily because they provide vitamins, minerals, and other substances important to good health. Data suggests that consuming a high-fiber diet (50 grams per day) may help to reduce glycemia, hyperinsulinemia, and lipemia in people with type 2 diabetes; however, gastrointestinal side effects such as gas, constipation, indigestion, and cramping can be potential barriers to achieving such a high fiber intake. Therefore, taking a first step of getting at least 14 grams per 1,000 calories can help alleviate some of those barriers. From there you can step up your intake gradually. Always drink plenty of water as you increase fiber intake as well, because this can help alleviate some side effects and keep the fiber moving smoothly through the digestive tract.

Your Nutrition Solution Tidbit: The market is loaded with fiber supplements, but if you want to get all of the benefits that fiber provides, don't take the easy way out. Whole foods provide more fiber as well as added essential nutrients such as vitamins, minerals, antioxidants, and phytonutrients that are necessary for optimal health. Never replace whole foods or any food group with a single simple supplement.

Sodium

Everyone should work to control the amount of sodium in their diet, but it is even more important for people with type 2 diabetes. Limiting the amount of sodium in your diet is key to helping prevent and/or manage high blood pressure, which can increase your risk for heart disease and stroke—two health issues for which people with type 2 diabetes are already at higher risk. You need some sodium in your diet because you need a certain balance of sodium and water in your body at all times for proper functioning, but too much salt or too much water will upset the balance. In a healthy person the kidneys get rid of extra sodium and fluids, helping to keep that balance. But too much sodium in your diet will eventually cause your body to retain or hold on to water, which puts an extra burden on your heart and blood vessels. In some people who are sodium sensitive this can lead to high blood pressure. Having less sodium in your diet can have the opposite effect and help to lower and/or avoid high blood pressure. Not everyone who eats too much sodium will end up with high blood pressure, according to the American Diabetes Association's Nutrition Principles and Recommendations in Diabetes, but people with type 2 diabetes are much more sensitive to the effects of sodium and therefore are at higher risk for high blood pressure, especially if they eat a high-sodium diet.

Table salt is made up of sodium and chloride. One teaspoon of table salt contains approximately 2,400 mg of sodium. Most of the sodium that people consume comes from processed and packaged foods, the worst of which are fast foods. Other foods high in sodium include canned soups and vegetables (with salt); condiments such as ketchup, cottage cheese, salad dressing, and canned sauces; pickled foods; processed meats such as lunch meat, bacon, sausage, hot dogs, and ham; olives;

salty snack foods; and monosodium glutamate (MSG), which is added to many foods as a preservative. Stick to foods that have a naturally lower sodium content such as fresh fruits and vegetables; fresh or frozen meats (no processed); dried beans, peas, and legumes; whole-grain foods prepared without salt; and unsalted nuts and seeds.

> **Your Nutrition Solution Tidbit:** If you are thinking of trying a salt substitute in place of table salt be aware that they can be very high in potassium, which can be dangerous for some people. Check with your doctor before adding these to your daily diet.

Here are some tips to help you decrease your sodium intake:

- Use fresh ingredients when cooking, and leave out the salt. Try using herbs and spices and even fresh-squeezed lemon for extra flavor. Cooked onion and minced garlic are great flavor enhancers. Avoid mixed seasonings and spice blends that contain salt, such as garlic salt. Make sure you read the labels.

- Avoid convenience foods such as boxed meals, frozen dinners, instant cereals, and canned gravies. Instead, get out the cookbook and make your own so that you have control over the amount of sodium in the dish.

- If you do eat frozen entrées, limit their frequency and choose those that contain less than 600 mg of sodium. (Check the nutrition facts label to choose meals with less sodium content.)

- Choose canned soups and vegetables whose labels dictate "no salt added."

⌘ Watch your portion size on condiments such as ketchup, salsa, soy sauce, and salad dressing. They can be loaded with sodium in even a small serving size. Try making your own salsa or salad dressing at home to cut back on the sodium.

⌘ Swap out high-sodium snacks such as chips and pretzels with healthier, low-sodium snacks such as fruit, dried fruit, unsalted nuts, or unsalted peanut butter.

⌘ Even some healthier foods like milk and whole-wheat bread have enough sodium that consuming large quantities can add up. If you are a person with diabetes, watch your portion sizes with all foods and read food labels carefully.

⌘ Remove the salt shaker from the table altogether. It will be less tempting to use.

⌘ Be aware of what sodium claims on food labels actually mean:

> ⌘ "Sodium-Free" or "Salt-Free": less than 5 mg of sodium per labeled serving

> ⌘ "Very Low Sodium"/"Very Low Salt": 35 mg or less of sodium per serving

> ⌘ "Low sodium" or "Low Salt": 140 mg or less of sodium per serving

> ⌘ "Reduced Sodium" or "Reduced Salt": at least 25 percent less sodium per serving than a similar product (not necessarily *low* in sodium, so check mg of sodium and percent daily value to be sure)

> ⌘ "Lightly Salted" or "Light in Sodium": at least 50 percent less sodium per serving than a similar product.

> ⌘ "No Added Salt" or "Unsalted": the food doesn't have any *extra* salt; it is not totally salt-free

❧ Read the nutrition facts panel to choose foods lower in sodium. After looking at the label and finding out exactly how many milligrams of sodium are in the product, take a look at the serving size. That amount of sodium is specifically for the serving size given. Next take a look at the percent daily value. This percentage will tell you how much sodium in that one serving size will take up of your whole day's allotment of 2,300 mg.

Once you begin removing excess sodium from your diet you will begin to really taste the natural flavors of foods again. Many of us are so used to the taste of saltiness that not having the sodium can make foods taste bland at first, but once you get your taste buds back you will appreciate more and more the wonderful natural flavors foods have to offer!

Your Nutrition Solution Tidbit: The Dietary Guidelines for Americans recommends that healthy individuals get no more than 2,300 mg of sodium daily. People with type 2 diabetes without high blood pressure can follow these guidelines as well. However, people with type 2 diabetes with high blood pressure should strive to get no more than 1,500 mg of sodium daily.

Cholesterol

When we talk about cholesterol, we are discussing both the cholesterol in foods and the cholesterol in our blood. Monitoring blood cholesterol levels for people with type 2 diabetes is just as important as keeping a close eye on blood glucose, A1C levels, and blood pressure. In fact, people with type 2 diabetes have the same risk for heart attack and stroke as someone who already has cardiovascular disease, because type 2 diabetes tends to lower HDL ("good") cholesterol levels and raise triglycerides and LDL ("bad") cholesterol levels in the blood. This common condition even has a name: *diabetic dyslipidemia*. With this condition you are at risk for premature coronary heart disease and atherosclerosis, in which the arteries become clogged with excess fat and other substances such as cholesterol. Several studies have shown a link between insulin resistance, a precursor to type 2 diabetes, and diabetic dyslipidemia, with this condition developing before diabetes is even diagnosed.[4]

On the diet side of things, cholesterol is a fat-like substance found mostly in animal foods such as meat, eggs, cheese, whole milk, and poultry. Not only do we get cholesterol from the foods we eat, but our liver actually produces all the cholesterol we need—*no* dietary cholesterol is needed. Cholesterol does play an important role in the body, but problems can occur when we consume it in excess. Our body needs cholesterol for major functions in the body, including making hormones, bile acids, and vitamin D. In addition, cholesterol is part of every body cell. The unused excess cholesterol gets stored as plaque in the arteries, increasing the risk for heart disease and stroke. Therefore, limiting dietary cholesterol as well as the "bad" fats that raise blood cholesterol (saturated fats and trans fats) is part of a heart-healthy equation that, again, is so important for people with type 2 diabetes. Shoot for no more than 300 mg of dietary cholesterol daily. If you already have heart disease that number should drop to 200 mg daily.

Here are some ways to lower the cholesterol in your diet and in your blood:

- Most meats contain similar amounts of cholesterol per serving; however, saturated fat can vary widely, and we know that this can raise cholesterol levels even more than cholesterol itself. So select lean cuts of meat with minimal visible fat. Lean cuts of beef include round, chuck, sirloin, and loin. Lean cuts of pork include tenderloin and loin chops.

- Buy "choice" or "select" grades.

- Select lean, or better yet, extra lean ground beef, and trim all visible fat from meat before cooking.

- Choose white-meat poultry and remove the skin before or after cooking and before eating. Cooking with the skin on can help keep the meat moist. If choosing ground poultry, look for packaging that states it is made from all white meat or that it is "extra lean."

- Choose fish two times or more per week, grilled, broiled, or baked rather than breaded and/or fried.

- Think about adding a few meatless meals to your week that include plant sources of protein such as grains, beans, vegetables, and soy foods.

- Use liquid vegetable oils such as canola, olive, or sunflower instead of solid fats such as butter, lard, or shortening.

- Substitute egg whites for whole eggs for meals or in recipes (replace each whole egg with two egg whites).

- Substitute fat-free or low-fat dairy products for whole-fat versions.

- Increase your fiber intake.

- Reach and maintain a healthy weight.

- Perform regular, moderate exercise. It can help you lose weight, which can directly impact your cholesterol and triglyceride levels in a good way. It can lower triglycerides and increase HDL levels, both of which can lower your risk for heart disease and stroke.

Cholesterol is carried in the blood throughout the body through lipoproteins. There are two types of lipoproteins:

1. **High-Density Lipoproteins (HDL)** are considered the "good" cholesterol because they help remove cholesterol from the body. The higher your blood HDL level the better.

2. **Low-Density Lipoproteins (LDL)** are considered the "bad" cholesterol because they can lead to a buildup of cholesterol in the arteries. The lower your blood LDL level the better.

Your Nutrition Solution Tidbit: Triglycerides are not cholesterol, but they are another type of fat in the blood that, In addition to cholesterol, needs to be monitored to ensure you lower your risk for heart disease and stroke.

Many factors can affect your blood cholesterol levels, including age, heredity, diet, body weight, exercise, certain medications, and certain medical conditions. Speak with your doctor about how often you should have your cholesterol and triglycerides checked and what numbers you should be aiming for. Cholesterol levels in the blood can also be affected by blood pressure and blood glucose. If you don't have these under control, your cholesterol numbers can be off too. They all work hand in hand to lower your risk for heart disease, stroke, and other serious health conditions.

In general, target levels for blood cholesterol and triglycerides, normally called a "lipid profile," are:

↘ **TOTAL cholesterol:** less than 200 is desirable, 200–239 is borderline high, and above 240 is high.

- **HDL cholesterol:** higher than 40 mg/dL for men and 50 mg/dL for women; the higher the HDL cholesterol the better for protecting against heart disease.

- **LDL cholesterol:** less than 100 mg/dL. According to the American Heart Association, if you have additional cardiovascular risk factors, your doctor may want your levels to be less than 70 mg/dL. A person with diabetes who lowers his LDL cholesterol levels can reduce heart disease complications by 20 to 50 percent.

- **Triglycerides:** less than 150 mg/dL. The main form of fat in the body, triglycerides come from the foods we eat and are made by the liver. High triglycerides contribute to a buildup of plaque in the lining of the arteries, leading to hardening of the arteries and reduced blood flow.

Your Nutrition Solution Tidbit: If you are not able to control blood cholesterol and triglyceride levels with diet and lifestyle alone, your doctor may prescribe cholesterol-lowering medications. Keep in mind that these medications are only effective if you are following a low-cholesterol diet and a healthy lifestyle.

Alcohol

Alcohol provides calories but not much nutritional value. You may have wondered if alcohol is off-limits if you have diabetes. If adults with diabetes choose to drink alcohol, the American Diabetes Association recommends limiting it to a moderate amount, which is one drink per day or fewer for women and two drinks per day or fewer for men. One alcoholic beverage is defined as 12 ounces of beer, 5 ounces of wine, or 1.5 ounces of distilled spirits. You do need to take a few precautions if you plan to partake in a few cocktails:

- Never drink on an empty stomach or if your blood sugar is low, especially if you are on insulin or oral medications.

- Alcohol should be considered an addition to a regular meal plan, and no food should be omitted to "fit the alcohol in."

- Keep a zero-calorie beverage with you (such as water), and drink that in addition to the alcohol to keep you hydrated.

- Stick to light beers and make a spritzer out of wine by adding ice and club soda.

- For mixed drinks, choose calorie-free mixers such as diet soft drinks, club soda, or other diet drinks.

- Don't let an alcoholic drink fuzz your judgement as to which foods you should and should not be eating.

- If you are drinking, do not drive!

The symptoms of too much alcohol and hypoglycemia (low blood sugar) can be quite similar, so be careful and don't mistake one for the other. Staying away from alcohol is strongly advised for people with a history of dependency problems, women who are pregnant or breastfeeding, and people with serious medical problems. Talk to your doctor if you are unsure as to whether moderate alcohol consumption is safe for you.

A Word on Herbs and Supplements

It can be tempting to try herbs and supplements that promise quick fixes and cures to your ailments. But be careful not to replace proven conventional medical treatment for type 2 diabetes with something that is unproven. There is currently no strong evidence that any specific herbal supplement can help to control diabetes or its complications, though research continues. Both dietary supplements and herbals can interact with medications as well as other supplements. If you are considering taking any type of herbal or dietary supplement, whether for diabetes or anything else, always talk to your doctor first.

chapter 3

your 5-step nutrition and lifestyle solution

What we put in our bodies nutritionally and how we treat our bodies physically can have a huge impact on our overall health—and on our type 2 diabetes. This chapter will discuss five important steps to follow that will help you manage your type 2 diabetes and decrease your risk for diabetes complications. Treatment for type 2 diabetes is very individualized, so it is important to do what works best for *you* and to get professional help from your doctor as well as a registered dietitian nutritionist (RDN) and/or a certified diabetes educator (CDE).

Generally speaking, doing physical activity, reaching a healthy weight, and having an overall better nutritional intake can help to control blood glucose levels and delay the progression of type 2 diabetes as well as prevent serious complications for most people with type 2 diabetes. The key is to empower yourself and to understand that even with support and education from your healthcare team, it is ultimately *you* who needs to make the changes. The best part is that all five of these steps are things you can control, and you can achieve all five goals on your own. It is exciting to realize that even though type 2 diabetes is a life-long disease for most, there *are* changes *you* can make to improve your health and your life.

Step 1: Reach and/or Maintain a Healthy Weight

Obesity is a known risk factor for type 2 diabetes. People who are overweight carry a much higher risk of developing type 2 diabetes than people who are at a healthy weight. The more fatty tissue you have, the tougher it is for the body to properly control your blood sugar using insulin, which causes insulin resistance. If you have diabetes and you are overweight or obese, losing just a small amount of weight can have a big impact on blood sugar control and help prevent serious complications due to type 2 diabetes as well. Just like modifying your eating and lifestyle behaviors and choosing an overall healthier diet, reaching and maintaining a healthy weight is within your control. The bottom line is that if you are overweight or obese you can help manage your diabetes by losing some of those unwanted pounds. As a bonus you will boost your overall health! If you are already at a healthy weight then the goal is to maintain that weight. If you are overweight or obese then the goal is to slowly and steadily lose weight in a healthy manner: no more than one or two pounds per week. Always check with your doctor first to discuss the weight-loss strategy that is best for you and to be thoroughly checked out before starting an appropriate weight-loss plan.

Determining Your Healthy Weight

Your first step is to get an idea of what your healthy weight is so that you have a smart goal in mind. Finding your BMI, or Body Mass Index, is one way to determine what your healthy weight is and whether any extra pounds translate into greater health risk. BMI is the measurement of your weight relative to your height, and can determine whether you are at a healthy weight or if your weight is possibly contributing to your type 2 diabetes. Keep in mind that BMI is not a measurement of body *fat*; therefore it can sometimes misclassify people. For example, someone with a lot of muscle mass may have a BMI that shows too high because BMI doesn't take into consideration that the majority of his or her body weight is coming from muscle rather than fat. It can do the opposite for elderly people and underestimate their BMI, not taking into account the muscle mass they have lost throughout the years. However, for the majority of us, our BMI is a good general indicator of our healthy weight range and whether we are putting our health at risk.

You can crunch the numbers yourself by using this formula:

Weight in pounds ÷ [height in inches]^2 x 703

You can also find calculators online, such as the one on ChooseMyPlate.gov (*www.choosemyplate.gov/supertracker-tools/resources/bmi-calculator.html*), or you can use the chart on pages

86 and 87 (intended for adults over 18 years of age) to easily find your BMI.

To use this BMI chart, locate your height in the left-hand column and follow the row across that height to find your weight. Follow the weight column up to the top to locate your BMI number.

Now that you know your BMI, what exactly does it mean? Healthy weight is a range, not one single weight. The following chart will show you what range you fall into and what your BMI means for you:

BMI	Weight
Below 18.5	Underweight
18.5 to 24.9	Healthy Weight
25.0 to 29.9	Overweight
Over 30.0	Obese

Your Nutrition Solution Tidbit: BMI for children and adolescents is determined differently. Because they are continually growing, their BMI is instead plotted on a growth chart. The percentile indicates the relative position of a child's BMI compared to that among children of the same gender and age.

Why Does My Body Shape Matter?

BMI is only one factor in assessing your weight. For an accurate assessment of weight related to health it is also important to look at *where* you store fat. As we discussed in an earlier chapter, the shape of our body, or where we store that excess fat, is compared to fruit: apples and pears.

- If you are shaped more like an apple, meaning you store and carry the majority of your fat in the stomach area and around your waist, you are at a higher risk for certain health problems such as cardiovascular disease, high blood pressure, type 2 diabetes, and certain types of cancer. Because type 2 diabetes already puts you at risk for heart disease, being overweight and carrying it in these areas increases your risk even more.

- If you are shaped more like a pear, meaning you store and carry the majority of your fat below the waist, in your hips, buttocks, and thighs, your shape does not put you at as much of a health risk as storing fat in other regions. This doesn't mean you don't need to drop that extra weight—those extra pounds are still causing more insulin resistance and making it tougher to control blood sugar. But the good news is it doesn't put you at a double risk for health issues related to weight, including heart disease.

Most of us are painfully aware of where we store every little bit of fat, so you shouldn't have much problem figuring out which fruit you resemble. But if you just can't decide whether you look more like an apple or a pear you can use your waist-to-hip ratio. Your waist-to-hip ratio can help determine, in a more scientific way, whether the location of your body fat is putting you at an even greater risk for health problems related to your weight.

BMI	19	20	21	22	23	24	25	26	27	28	29	30	31	32	33	34	35
Height								Weight in Pounds									
4'10"	91	96	100	105	110	115	119	124	129	134	138	143	148	153	158	162	167
4'11"	94	99	104	109	114	119	124	128	133	138	143	148	153	158	163	168	173
5'	97	102	107	112	118	123	128	133	138	143	148	153	158	163	168	174	179
5'1"	100	106	111	116	122	127	132	137	143	148	153	158	164	169	174	180	185
5'2"	104	109	115	120	126	131	136	142	147	153	158	164	169	175	180	186	191
5'3"	107	113	118	124	130	135	141	146	152	158	163	169	175	180	186	191	197
5'4"	110	116	122	128	134	140	145	151	157	163	169	174	180	186	192	197	204
5'5"	114	120	126	132	138	144	150	156	162	168	174	180	186	192	198	204	210
5'6"	118	124	130	136	142	148	155	161	167	173	179	186	192	198	204	210	216
5'7"	121	127	134	140	146	153	159	166	172	178	185	191	198	204	211	217	223

Height																	
5'8"	125	131	138	144	151	158	164	171	177	184	190	197	203	210	216	223	230
5'9"	128	135	142	149	155	162	169	176	182	189	196	203	209	216	223	230	236
5'10"	132	139	146	153	160	167	174	181	188	195	202	209	216	222	229	236	243
5'11"	136	143	150	157	165	172	179	186	193	200	208	215	222	229	236	243	250
6'	140	147	154	162	169	177	184	191	199	206	213	221	228	235	242	250	258
6'1"	144	151	159	166	174	182	189	197	204	212	219	227	235	242	250	257	265
6'2"	148	155	163	171	179	186	194	202	210	218	225	233	241	249	256	264	272
6'3"	152	160	168	176	184	192	200	208	216	224	232	240	248	256	264	272	279
6'4"	156	164	172	180	189	197	205	213	221	230	238	246	254	263	271	279	287
	Healthy Weight						Overweight					Obese					

Source: *Evidence Report of Clinical Guidelines on the Identification, Evaluation, and Treatment of Overweight and Obesity in Adults, 1998. NIH/National Heart, Lung, and Blood Institute (NHLBI). Check out www.nhlbi.nih. gov/guidelines/obesity/bmi_tbl.htm for additional heights and weights.*

Follow these steps to figure out your waist-to-hip ratio:

1. Stand relaxed. Measure your waist at its smallest point, without sucking in your stomach or pulling the tape measure too tight.

2. Measure your hips by measuring the largest part of your buttocks and hips.

3. Divide your waist measurement by your hip measurement.

4. If this number is nearly or more than 1.0, you would be considered an apple shape.

5. If this number is considerably less than 1.0, you would be considered a pear shape.

Steps to Reaching a Healthy Weight

There are so many reasons to reach a healthy weight, and if you are reading this book, trying to manage your type 2 diabetes successfully and for the long term is probably at the top of your list. If you have a ways to go to get to your healthy weight range, take heart in knowing that a little bit can go a long way. If you are on the overweight side of the coin, losing just 10 pounds can be the ticket to improving your health and to begin improving blood sugar levels. But don't stop there! Reaching your healthy weight once and for all will not only help to better control your blood sugar, but it may also help you to avoid using oral medications and even insulin, so that you are ultimately able to manage your disease through diet and lifestyle changes alone. In addition, reaching a healthier weight will decrease your risk for the serious complications that go along with type 2 diabetes. Aside from the diabetes itself, reaching a healthier weight will end up helping in ways you never even considered.

If you are like most people, you want to lose weight the quickest and easiest way possible. Who doesn't? But resist the urge to sign up for fad diets or *any* type of "diet" that promises quick and easy weight loss. These types of diets usually revolve around deprivation of some type, and that can easily deplete your body's stores of essential, healthy nutrients. These types of diets are not healthy for anyone, but they can be downright dangerous to people with type 2 diabetes. They can spin blood sugars out of control and create risky situations. Furthermore, fast weight loss is usually the weight loss that never sticks. Also steer clear of liquid diets, diet pills, or diet supplements that promise that tempting quick fix. These can also be very dangerous, especially to a diabetic, and can include high levels of sugar. Slow and steady wins the race to long-lasting weight loss, better health, and improved blood sugar control. Losing just one to two pounds per week is a safe and effective goal. The ultimate goal is to incorporate a healthy diet that will allow you to lose weight into your overall diabetes management plan.

It doesn't take as much change as you think to begin losing weight. Making healthier choices by eliminating unhealthy foods and replacing them with healthier foods will, most of the time, automatically cut your calorie intake and make more of a change than you think. The idea is that for permanent weight loss you want to lose weight slowly, steadily, and in a healthy manner. Again, it doesn't take a whole lot to begin reversing the process and getting yourself on track. Worrying less about every little calorie and concentrating more in general on eating nutrient-rich foods that make calories count while still keeping an eye on your portion sizes will help control your calorie intake much better. This will ensure that even though you are trying to lose weight, you will still be getting all the essential nutrients your body needs for good health.

It is time to change bad habits into good ones, and that goes for eating as well as exercise. Here are a few steps to help you get started and thinking in the right direction for a healthy weight loss:

1. Your first order of business should be to think deeply about your true reasons for wanting to lose weight. Because you are reading this book it is a good bet that better managing your type 2 diabetes without the need for medications and/or insulin will be somewhere on that list. Knowing exactly what will motivate you and keep you committed to your goals is what will ultimately make you successful in your endeavor.

2. Secondly you need to set both short-term and long-term goals. You can't expect to transform your body overnight—that is a recipe for failure. Instead, set small, realistic, specific, and measurable goals for yourself. Once you have mastered one goal and it becomes habit, move on to the next. Write your goals down, along with your motivations, so you always know what you are working toward. For people with type 2 diabetes, changing eating habits are not only necessary for weight loss but also vital for blood sugar control and ultimately your health, so keep that in mind.

3. Keep a daily food diary that includes what you eat, when you eat, and how much you eat. Use this food diary to monitor your blood sugar as well. This will give you a chance to see how eating more healthily will improve these levels. Don't just write in your diary; review it frequently so that you can pinpoint and work on problem areas. Keeping a food diary will help to keep you compliant and on track.

4. Get in the habit of being aware of every food and beverage you put in your mouth. Make yourself accountable

for what you eat and the way you live your life. This will need to be a habit you get used to as a person with diabetes. But soon enough it will become second nature.

5. It is important to get support not just from an RDN and/or CDE but from others who may be going through the same journey you are. Connecting with others can provide you with emotional support when you feel like giving up. You can find a weight-loss buddy, join an online support group, or do whatever works for you.

Now that you are ready to go, here are some general strategies to help you begin losing weight in a healthy manner that is safe for those with type 2 diabetes. It is essential to speak with your doctor, RDN, and/or CDE before getting started on any type of weight loss plan. They can help direct and monitor you as well as individualize a plan for you.

>   Never skip meals—that includes breakfast! The most effective diet for people with type 2 diabetes is one that includes a healthy breakfast. You won't save calories by skipping, because skipping any meal will lead to eating more than you should at the next meal or cause uncontrolled snacking throughout the day—both of which will pack on more calories than you need and cause blood sugar levels to surge. Eating breakfast, especially if it is a whole-grain cereal, is associated with better weight loss and blood sugar control.

>   You need to cut back on calories to lose weight, but for people with type 2 diabetes that exact calorie level will depend on age, gender, current weight, activity level, body type, and current blood sugar control. In general, a reasonable goal is between 1,200 and 1,800 calories per day for women and between 1,400 and 2,000 calories per day for men. Your RDN and/or CDE can help

you to personalize this goal and provide you with a calorie range that will help you to achieve weight loss while properly managing your blood sugar levels.

⅍ Don't count each and every calorie you eat as a way of keeping track. That can become tedious and time consuming. Instead use ChooseMyPlate.gov to get an idea of how many servings of each food group you need daily in order to stick to your calorie level and how big those serving sizes should be. This will be a much easier way to stick to a certain calorie level. You will need to combine this with carb counting at each meal, which we will discuss later in this chapter.

⅍ Stick to a well-balanced and healthy eating routine. Healthier choices usually mean fewer calories, less fat, less sodium, and more nutritional value. The USDA's Dietary Guidelines for Americans can provide you with information on good dietary habits, which we will discuss later in this chapter.

⅍ Cut back on or cut out junk foods such as candy, cookies, cake, pies, other sweets, soft drinks, fast foods, and chips. This is not only a must for weight loss but for good blood sugar control as well. Switch from these foods to healthier snacks. Your RDN and/or CDE can help you fit a few goodies into your plan on occasion.

⅍ Plan your healthy meals and snacks ahead of time so that you are always prepared. Having what you need at work or at home is key to eating the right foods. Not being prepared is what can get you into trouble.

⅍ Be diligent with portion control. Sticking to correct portion sizes will help with weight loss and with managing blood sugar levels.

⅍ Avoid eating in front of the television (especially late-night snacks) or computer or while doing other activities that keep you from paying attention to what you are eating and how much you are eating.

- Get in the habit of slowing yourself down while eating. It takes a good 20 minutes for your brain to get the message that you are full. Eating too quickly leads to overeating, which can lead to excess weight and possibly quicker spikes in blood sugar.

- Use a smaller plate to dish up your food. It will help to keep your portions and calories under control and make you feel that you are getting a full plate of food. Just don't go back for seconds!

- Plan and prepare more meals at home to keep from eating out too often. You don't have to be a chef to do this. Invest in some healthy cookbooks, look for recipes online, or share recipes with friends. Restaurant meals tend to be higher in calories and fat, and it can be too difficult to make the right choices when eating out. Don't deprive yourself of eating out, but make it an occasional outing instead of a regular habit, and work on making better choices when you do.

- Learn how to read and use the Nutrition Facts Panel on food labels to your advantage. The Nutrition Facts Panel can help you to choose foods that best fit into your goals. It provides a measurement of portion sizes, carbohydrates, calories, and other essential nutrients. (We will discuss more about food labels in Chapter 5.)

- Check out the USDA's ChooseMyPlate.gov site to explore all of the information and hands-on tools that can help you lose weight sensibly and at the same time teach you what good nutrition really means.

- Incorporate some type of physical activity most days of the week. Overweight and obesity is a direct result of an imbalance between the calories you take in and the calories you burn. It is just that simple. The more active you are, the more calories you will burn. Something as simple as walking can be a great start. We will discuss exercise in detail later in this chapter.

ℵ Drink plenty of water throughout each day. Staying properly hydrated is essential to digestion and the fat-burning process.

ℵ Include plenty of fiber in your daily diet. We already know fiber can help you better manage blood sugar levels, but it can also help with weight loss. High-fiber meals and snacks help fill you up and keep you feeling fuller longer. Go back to Chapter 2 for tips on increasing you fiber intake.

These tips and changes can help you improve your health, lose weight, and control your type 2 diabetes. It is all about making permanent lifestyle changes that you can and will stick with for a lifetime. Once you begin to lose weight, feel better, and experience how much easier it is to control and manage your type 2 diabetes, you will be motivated to push ahead and continue your journey. Once you reach your weight goal, don't go back to your old ways. The next step is to maintain your new healthy weight and keep your new healthy habits as part of your lifestyle.

2. Control Your Carbohydrate Intake

We discussed the importance of carbohydrates, especially for people with type 2 diabetes in Chapter 2. Carbohydrates affect blood sugar, so you need to control how many and when you eat them for effective diabetic meal planning. Your daily carb allowance will depend on your weight, your weight-loss goals, how active you are, your age, any medical conditions you have, and what, if any, medication you take. People who are active on a regular basis can usually eat a few more carbs and still keep blood sugar levels controlled. Finding the correct balance for you is important so that you can feel your best and have the energy to do the things you want to do while keeping diabetic complications to a minimum. Your RDN and/or CDE can calculate exactly how many carbs you should be consuming daily, but a good general start is 45 to 60 grams of carbs per meal, with about 15 to 30 grams for between-meal snacks. Carbohydrates should generally provide somewhere between 45 and 60 percent of your daily total calories. And don't forget the other components of your diet, which are proteins and fats. They will not affect blood sugar directly, but are still an important part of a complete and healthy diet.

For example, if your calorie needs are 2,000 per day, your carb needs would be between 900 and 1,200 calories:

$$2{,}000 \times [0.45 \text{ to } 0.60] = 900 \text{ to } 1200 \text{ calories}$$
$$\text{coming from carbohydrates}$$

There are four calories per gram of carb, so if your calorie needs are 2,000 calories, you have approximately 225 to 300 grams of carbs to space evenly throughout the day. Of course this depends on other factors as well, but this is a general example to explain how it works:

$$900 \text{ to } 1200 \div 4 = 225 \text{ to } 300 \text{ grams of}$$
$$\text{carbohydrates for a 2,000-calorie diet}$$

Figure out Your Calorie Needs

Calorie needs depend on many factors, such as age, height, weight, muscle mass, activity level, gender, and, for women, whether they are pregnant. In other words, calorie needs are very individualized. Your best bet is to get a true number from your CDE and/or RDN. However, to get a general idea you can use the chart on pages 98 and 99. First, choose the statement out of the following list that best describes your activity level:

1. **Not Active:** I don't do anything more than I need to do for my usual activities of work, school, chores, cleaning, shopping, and so on.

2. **Moderately active:** I do some moderate exercise daily in addition to doing my usual activities. For example, I briskly walk one to three miles daily or something similar.

3. **Very active:** I am very active every day in addition to my usual activities. I briskly walk or jog three or more miles daily or something similar.

Now find the line on the chart that applies to your age, gender, and level of activity. Remember that this chart is only an estimation of how many calories your body needs to maintain the weight it is at right now.

Note: Estimates are rounded to the nearest 200 calories. An individual's calorie needs may be higher or lower than these average estimates.

Your Nutrition Solution Tidbit: About 3,500 calories add up to one pound. Therefore, to lose one pound per week you need to split up a deficit of 3,500 calories over a week's time. Deducting 500 calories per day should result in a one-pound-per-week weight loss.

What Foods Contain Carbohydrates?

Foods that contain carbohydrates include grains such as oats, oatmeal, barley, and rice; grain-based foods such as breads, pastas, cereals, and crackers; starchy vegetables such as corn, peas, and potatoes (other vegetables have carbs as well but very little); fruits and fruit juices; milk, yogurt, and other dairy products; dried beans and lentils; and most sweets and snack foods. Basically most foods, other than meats and fats, contain some amount of carbohydrates. It is important to realize that all types of carbohydrates, whether they are found in a piece of bread or a piece of candy, will raise blood sugar levels. Maybe at different rates, but eventually all carbs are converted into glucose in the body. For example, a brownie could have 30 grams of carbohydrates and that brownie will raise blood glucose the same as 2/3 cup of rice, which also has 30 grams of carbohydrates.

Adding "Free" Foods

Certain foods are considered "free" foods because when they are consumed in specified portions, they do not need to be added to your total carbohydrate allowance for the day. Free foods have very little impact on blood sugar levels, and include anything that contains 5 grams or less of carbs and fewer than 20 calories. Certain free foods should be limited to no more than three servings per day, and spread throughout the day. These free foods include sauces, salsa, fat-free or low-fat condiments, low-fat or fat-free salad dressing, fat-free or low-fat sour cream or cream cheese, and pickles. Although these are considered "free" foods you still need to be aware of the portion size you are eating to ensure it is still considered a "free" food. Other "free" foods that have even less impact on blood sugar

Gender/Activity Level	Male/Sedentary	Male/Moderately Active	Male/Active	Female/Sedentary	Female/Moderately Active	Female/Active
Age (years)						
2	1,000	1,000	1,000	1,000	1,000	1,000
3	1,200	1,400	1,400	1,000	1,200	1,400
4	1,200	1,400	1,600	1,200	1,400	1,400
5	1,200	1,400	1,600	1,200	1,400	1,600
6	1,400	1,600	1,800	1,200	1,400	1,600
7	1,400	1,600	1,800	1,200	1,600	1,800
8	1,400	1,600	2,000	1,400	1,600	1,800
9	1,600	1,800	2,000	1,400	1,600	1,800
10	1,600	1,800	2,200	1,400	1,800	2,000
11	1,800	2,000	2,200	1,600	1,800	2,000
12	1,800	2,200	2,400	1,600	2,000	2,200
13	2,000	2,200	2,600	1,600	2,000	2,200
14	2,000	2,400	2,800	1,800	2,000	2,400

Age						
15	2,200	2,600	3,000	1,800	2,000	2,400
16	2,400	2,800	3,200	1,800	2,000	2,400
17	2,400	2,800	3,200	1,800	2,000	2,400
18	2,400	2,800	3,200	1,800	2,000	2,400
19-20	2,600	2,800	3,000	2,000	2,200	2,400
21-25	2,400	2,800	3,000	2,000	2,200	2,400
26-30	2,400	2,600	3,000	1,800	2,000	2,400
31-35	2,400	2,600	3,000	1,800	2,000	2,200
36-40	2,400	2,600	2,800	1,800	2,000	2,200
41-45	2,200	2,600	2,800	1,800	2,000	2,200
46-50	2,200	2,400	2,800	1,800	2,000	2,200
51-55	2,200	2,400	2,800	1,600	1,800	2,200
56-60	2,200	2,400	2,600	1,600	1,800	2,200
61-65	2,000	2,400	2,600	1,600	1,800	2,000
66-70	2,000	2,200	2,600	1,600	1,800	2,000
71-75	2,000	2,200	2,600	1,600	1,800	2,000
76+	2,000	2,200	2,400	1,600	1,800	2,000

Source: Developed from the 2010 Dietary Guidelines for Americans and Diabetes.org.

and can be eaten with a little less restriction include broth, club soda, diet soft drinks, sugar-free gelatin, flavored water (no sugar), lemon juice, sugar substitutes, hot sauce, horserad-ish, and unsweetened tea and coffee.

Carbohydrate Counting

The key to controlling carbohydrate intake is to spread your allotment of carbs (both sugars and starches) evenly through-out the day and to keep your eating schedule consistent from day to day. Although carbs are basically the only nutrient in food that directly affects blood sugar, you also need to balance your meals with an appropriate amount of lean protein and healthy fats. Carb counting is a method that is used for diabetes meal planning and is a fairly simple way to balance and to keep track of the amount of total carbohydrates you eat each day. It gives you a bit more flexibility and variety in food choices, allowing you to eat more of what you want.

> **Your Nutrition Solution Tidbit:** The Nutrition Facts Panel on packaged foods lists total carbohydrates, which includes sugars, starches, dietary fiber, and sugar alcohols. Because fiber is a type of carbohy-drate that the body does not digest, it really does not affect your blood sugar levels. You can subtract the grams of fiber from the total carbohydrate amount before counting those carbohydrates into your diet plan.

Counting grams of carbs along with evenly distributing them in your meals and snacks should help to control your blood sugar levels.

Knowing how many grams of carbohydrates are in one serving of a carb-related food and the fact that one carbohydrate serving is equal to 15 grams of carbohydrates is all you need to know to count carbs. If you eat more carbs than your insulin supply can handle, your blood sugar level will go up. If you eat too few, your blood sugar can fall too low. You can manage these fluctuations by knowing how to count your carbohydrate intake.

An RDN and/or CDE can help you to figure out a plan for carb counting that meets your specific needs, but in general, for adults, a typical plan usually includes three to four servings of carbohydrates at each meal and one to two carbohydrate servings at each snack. When you use the method of carb counting to manage blood sugar, you can choose just about any food product (healthier ones more often) as long as you know how many carbs it has per serving. The Nutrition Facts Panel on packaged foods provides you with information on grams of carbohydrates per serving so that you are able to fit the food into your type 2 diabetes meal plan. But look carefully at serving size, because you need to eat that exact amount to get the amount of carbs listed. Adjust the serving size accordingly to get only the carbohydrates you need. Carb counting can work for just about any person with type 2 diabetes, whether they manage blood glucose with diet alone or they use oral medication and/or insulin. It takes some pre-planning when you get started, but the more you work with this method, the better you will become at knowing the amount of carbs in foods. It will be helpful at first to monitor your blood sugars before and after meals and snacks to see where adjustments need to be made.

Here are a few examples of what 15 grams of carbohydrates looks like:

- 1 small piece of fresh fruit
- 1 slice of bread

- ⋈ 1 6-inch tortilla
- ⋈ 1/2 cup oatmeal
- ⋈ 1/3 cup pasta or rice, cooked
- ⋈ 1/2 English muffin or hamburger bun
- ⋈ 1/2 cup beans or a starchy vegetable
- ⋈ 3 oz. baked potato
- ⋈ 2/3 cup yogurt, plain, fat-free
- ⋈ 1 cup soup
- ⋈ 1/2 cup casserole

You can check out the following online document for a full list of what would count as 15 grams of carbohydrates: *http://dtc.ucsf.edu/pdfs/FoodLists.pdf.*

> **Your Nutrition Solution Tidbit:** Don't stockpile your carbs. In other words, you don't "save up" the carbs you didn't eat for breakfast and lunch so that you can use them at dinner. Unfortunately it doesn't work that way. This causes imbalances in your carb intake that will show in your blood glucose levels. You need to spread carbs evenly throughout the day for good control.

It is a smart idea to keep some type of simple food diary, not only to help you keep track of your carbohydrate intake but also to make you are more aware of your eating patterns. Keep a diary until you are confident in your ability to control your blood sugar and carb counts. Write down everything you eat and drink as well as portion sizes. You can also use your food diary to keep track of blood sugar levels. This way you have information to use to make necessary adjustments to your meal plan. You can bring the diary to share at your appointments with your doctor, RDN, and/or CDE so that you are all on the same page.

On the next page I've given an example of a good food diary.

When you are using a carb-counting method, serving size is everything. Do not be tempted, especially when first starting out, to eyeball or guesstimate your portion sizes and food measurements. Use measuring cups and spoons as well as a food scale so you know for a fact exactly what your portion sizes are. You may be surprised at the difference between guessing and actually measuring! Overestimating or underestimating your portion sizes can completely throw your blood sugar levels off and make carb counting a lot more frustrating than it needs to be. Carbohydrate counting, as with any new skill, takes practice. Measuring your foods will help you improve your confidence and accuracy.

Your Nutrition Solution Tidbit: Sugar alcohols can be found in products that are labeled as "sugar free" or "no sugar added." The effect of these sugar alcohols on blood sugar is less than regular sugar or glucose. Because only about half of sugar alcohols are absorbed, only count half of the sugar alcohol, if it is stated on a label, as a carbohydrate when carb counting. Sugar alcohols can be harder for the body to digest, and eating too many can result in digestive problems such as gas, cramping, and diarrhea. Examples of sugar alcohols are sorbitol, xylitol, mannitol, isomalt, maltitol, lactitol, and hydrogenated starch hydrolysates.

3. Follow a Healthy Plate

Following a healthy plate has a double meaning for people with type 2 diabetes. We are going to discuss not only putting healthier foods on your plate but also a simple method called the "Healthy Plate" method to keep your diet on track and your blood sugar levels steady.

The Healthy Plate method is a good starting point for people with type 2 diabetes, and it can also help you jump-start weight loss or maintain a healthy weight. It can also be a good long-term method to stick with in addition to carb counting to always remind you of how you should be eating for better blood glucose control. Following the Healthy Plate method allows you to choose the foods you want to eat but changes the portion sizes you are eating.

Follow these steps to initiate the Healthy Plate method:

- Start with an ordinary dinner plate. Put a line down the middle of your plate, either real or imaginary. Then divide one side in half so that you end up with 3 sections on your plate.

- Fill the largest section with non-starchy vegetables such as spinach, carrots, broccoli, cauliflower, tomatoes, mushrooms, zucchini, or asparagus.

- Fill one of the smaller sections on the opposite side of the plate with grains and/or starchy vegetables such as whole-wheat bread, whole-grain cereal, brown rice, whole-grain pasta, cooked beans, oatmeal, potatoes, corn, sweet potatoes, winter squash, popcorn, or pretzels.

- Fill the remaining section with a lean protein source such as lean beef, skinless chicken or turkey breast, pork loin, fish, eggs, tofu, or low-fat cheese.

> ⅃ Add a serving of fruit and/or fat-free or low-fat dairy, depending on your individualized meal plan.

> ⅃ To complete the meal you can add one to two servings of a healthy fat such as salad dressing or olive oil to vegetables, or a few slices of avocado to a sandwich.

Once you begin to master portion and carb control, you can begin to work on choosing healthier food options from each food group. As important as it is to count carbs to control blood sugar, it is just as important to eat a healthier diet to ward off other health issues. The good news is that you have a wealth of nutrition information on how to eat and live more healthily right at your fingertips. That information is the USDA's ChooseMyPlate.gov and the Dietary Guidelines for Americans. Reading them is the perfect first step to help you make healthier nutritional and lifestyle choices in order to begin better managing your type 2 diabetes.

Your Nutrition Solution Tidbit: Both ChooseMyPlate .gov and the Dietary Guidelines for Americans are issued and updated jointly by the Department of Agriculture (USDA) and the Department of Health and Human Services (HHS) every five years. The guidelines work hand in hand to provide the most current science-based advice for all Americans aged 2 years and older. They are available for all Americans so that we can educate ourselves as to what good nutrition is and how we can make healthier choices. The key is not to only read both of these educational components but also to implement them in your everyday life.

My Type 2 Diabetes Diary					
Time/ Meal	Blood Sugar Level	Medi- cation and/or Insulin Dose	Food/ Beverage Intake & Amount	Total Grams of Carbs	
Break- fast					
Snack					
Lunch					Comments
Snack					
Dinner					
Snack					

ChooseMyPlate.gov

ChooseMyPlate.gov is a fairly new Website that showcases the newer MyPlate icon, which took the place of the Food

Guide Pyramid in 2010. MyPlate works hand in hand with the Dietary Guidelines for Americans to help all people:

⊠ Make smarter choices from each food group

⊠ Find a healthy balance between food and physical activity

⊠ Get the most nutrition out of calories consumed

⊠ Stay within daily calorie needs

The MyPlate icon emphasizes the five food groups, which are the foundation of a healthy diet, by dividing the familiar dinner plate into four sections for fruits, vegetables, grains, and proteins, with a fifth, smaller place to one side for dairy foods. MyPlate illustrates these food groups as separate colors and different sizes on the plate. For example, the fruit (red) and vegetable (green) portions make up half of the plate to emphasize the recommendation that you should include fruits and vegetables as at least half of every meal. MyPlate is only slightly different from the Healthy Plate method we spoke about first. The only difference is on the half section of the plate, MyPlate contains both fruits and vegetables, whereas the Healthy Plate method contains only non-starchy vegetables, with a piece of fruit and/or dairy on the side. Still, they follow the same concept: filling your plate with healthier foods and including all of the food groups is key to better health. All of the healthy recommendations for the general public from MyPlate can be used for people with type 2 diabetes as well. Key suggestions for the MyPlate guide include:

Food to Increase:

⊠ Fill half your plate with fruits and vegetables

⊠ Switch to fat-free or low-fat (1%) milk

⊠ Make at least half of your grains whole grains

⊠ Go lean with protein sources

Foods to Reduce:

- Compare the sodium (salt) in foods like soup, bread, and frozen meals, and choose foods with lower numbers
- Drink water instead of sugary drinks

Balancing Calories:

- Enjoy your food, but eat less
- Avoid oversized portions
- Find a balance between food and physical activity

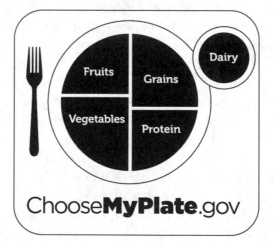

In addition to the MyPlate icon, ChooseMyPlate.gov is full of helpful tools to start you on the path to a healthier diet. The Website includes:

- **MyPlate:** This section dives into each food group included in the MyPlate Icon in detail and provides you with all of the information you need to make healthier selections from each group.
- **Weight Management and Calories:** This section is dedicated to helping you understand how calories are related to weight loss.

⊁ **Physical Activity:** This section provides you with important information on physical activity and how to use it to your advantage.

⊁ **SuperTracker and Other Tools:** The SuperTracker is a tool to help you plan, analyze, and track your diet as well as your physical activity. Other helpful tools in this section include Calories Burn Chart, Calories Count Chart for Mixed Dishes, Empty Calories Chart, Solids Fat Chart, BMI Calculator, Portion Distortion, and Food Labeling. There is also a Food-A-Pedia that gives you access to 8,000-plus foods and their nutrition info. This is a great place to look up carbohydrate contents of foods for carb counting.

This Website has all of the information and more that you need to start eating a healthier diet. And if you think that eating a healthier diet isn't part of the solution to managing your type 2 diabetes, you would be very wrong! Try it and find out just how much it helps!

Source: USDA ChooseMyPlate.gov, www.choosemyplate.gov

The Dietary Guidelines for Americans

The newest set of Dietary Guidelines for Americans focuses on three major goals that together emphasize a total lifestyle approach:

1. Balance calories with physical activity to manage weight.

2. Consume more healthy foods and nutrients such as fruits, vegetables, whole grains, fat-free and low-fat dairy products, and seafood.

3. Consume fewer foods with sodium (salt), saturated fats, trans fats, cholesterol, added sugars, and refined grains.

These guidelines are intended to aide Americans in maintaining a healthy weight, reducing the risk of chronic disease, and promoting overall good health. The current Dietary Guidelines for Americans include 23 specific key recommendations for the general population and six additional key recommendations for specific groups whose needs may differ slightly, such as pregnant women. These recommendations are meant to help you reach the three major goals set by the guidelines. In the following lists I will summarize the 23 general recommendations, but I highly encourage you to visit *www.cnpp.usda.gov/ DietaryGuidelines.htm* to read the full guidelines. They are key to adopting healthier lifestyle habits that will help manage your type 2 diabetes, reduce your risk for numerous chronic diseases, and increase your chances for living a longer, healthier life. It is all up to you!

Balancing Calories to Manage Weight

1. **Prevent and/or reduce overweight and obesity through improved eating and physical activity behaviors.** These are lifestyle changes *you* have control over that will help you to manage not only your weight and your health but also your blood sugar levels and complications from type 2 diabetes.

2. **Control total calorie intake to manage body weight. For people who are overweight or obese, this will mean consuming fewer calories from foods and beverages.** Balancing your calorie intake over time is the key to weight management and keeping weight off long term. This means balancing the calories you burn

through physical activity with the number of calories you consume. If these numbers are equal, you will maintain your weight; if they shift to the negative, you will lose weight; if they shift to the positive, ultimately you will gain weight. So the goal here is to gain control over this balance of calories in and calories out and shift it in your favor.

3. **Increase physical activity and reduce time spent in sedentary behaviors.** Physical activity has all types of health and even mental benefits, and it is essential in the calorie balance equation for weight management. (We will discuss exercise later in this chapter.)

4. **Maintain appropriate calorie balance during each stage of life—childhood, adolescence, adulthood, pregnancy and breastfeeding, and older age.** Maintaining the calorie-in and calorie-out equation should not be a temporary situation to lose weight; it should be a lifelong adjustment to maintain your healthy weight. It is much easier to balance this equation and maintain your healthy weight than it is to gain weight and then have to lose it. Lifestyle and eating habits need to change permanently in order to maintain a healthy weight and improved health.

Foods and Food Components to Reduce

5. **Reduce daily sodium intake to less than 2,300 milligrams (mg); persons who are 51 and older and those of any age who are African American or have hypertension, diabetes, or chronic kidney disease must further reduce intake to 1,500 mg. The 1,500 mg recommendation applies to about half of the U.S. population, including children and adults.** Most

Americans consume way more sodium than what is recommended and what our bodies need. On average, Americans consume around 3,400 milligrams per day. Research from the American Heart Association has indicated that as sodium levels decrease, so does blood pressure. When our blood pressure is in the normal range we decrease our risk for cardiovascular disease, kidney disease, and congestive heart failure—all three of which people with type 2 diabetes are at higher risk for.

6. **Consume less than 10 percent of calories from saturated fats by replacing them with monounsaturated and polyunsaturated fatty acids.** Added fats come with loads of calories that you don't need, and choosing the wrong types of fat too often can cause a host of health problems such as heart disease, stroke, and high cholesterol.

7. **Consume less than 300 mg per day of dietary cholesterol.** We need cholesterol in our bodies for a few essential functions, but our body makes more than enough for these specific purposes. Therefore we need very little in the way of cholesterol-containing foods in our daily diet. Too much dietary cholesterol in our diet can lead to high levels of LDL (or the "bad" cholesterol), which in turn can lead to cardiovascular disease and stroke.

8. **Keep trans fatty acid consumption as low as possible, especially by limiting foods that contain synthetic sources of trans fats such as partially hydrogenated oils, and by limiting other solid fats.** Trans fats are unsaturated fats, but they differ in their structure from other unsaturated fats and therefore are not considered healthy as are the other unsaturated fats. Trans fats are not essential in our diets. They can be found naturally

in some foods and formed during processing (hydrogenation) in others. It is the trans fats that are formed during processing that tend to be the most damaging to our health. To find trans fats in foods check the food label and look for the words "hydrogenated oil" or "partially hydrogenated oil" in the ingredient list.

9. **Reduce the intake of calories from solid fats and added sugars.** The American Heart Association tells us that the intake of saturated fats and trans fats can increase our risk for chronic disease, especially cardiovascular disease. Most fats with a high percentage of saturated and trans fats are solid at room temperature and therefore are referred to as "solid fats." Sugar can be found naturally in some foods, including lactose in most dairy products and fructose in fruits. However, the majority of sugars found in the average American diet are added sugars. These sugars are added in processing, preparation, or at the table to sweeten and improve palatability. They are also added as a preservative and to provide texture, body, viscosity, and browning capacity to foods. Although our body cannot determine the difference between natural and added sugars, foods with natural sugars usually contain the whole package of nutrients and other healthful components such as fiber, whereas most foods with added sugars often supply calories with little to no essential nutrients and no fiber. Solid fats and added sugars are a particular concern in the American diet because both have been found to be consumed in excessive amounts. Together, these two food components contribute a substantial number of calories to our diets—35 percent of total daily calories—without contributing to our nutritional needs. This makes them very dangerous when it comes

to managing weight. When consumed in excess, foods that contain solid fats and added sugars begin to take the place of foods with essential vitamins, minerals, and fiber. Reducing the consumption of these foods allows us to increase our intake of nutrient-dense foods without going over our total daily calorie needs.

Your Nutrition Solution Tidbit: The World Health Organization (WHO) recently drafted new guidelines stating that both added and naturally occurring sugars should make up less than 5 percent of a person's total caloric intake each day to help prevent obesity and tooth decay.[1]

10. **Limit the consumption of foods that contain refined grains, especially refined grain foods that contain solid fats, added sugars, and sodium.** The goal should be to eat at least half of your grains as whole grains and to limit refined grains, especially those that contain solid fats and added sugars.

11. **If alcohol is consumed, it should be consumed in moderation—up to one drink per day for women and two drinks per day for men—and only by adults of legal drinking age.** As reported in the Guidelines, approximately 50 percent of American adults are regular drinkers, with 29 percent reporting that they occasionally binge drink. The consumption of alcohol can have beneficial effects or detrimental effects depending on how much is consumed and how often, as well as a person's age and health issues. Alcohol consumption may have beneficial effects when consumed in moderation, especially red wine. However, it is never recommended

to start drinking if you are a non-drinker. Excessive drinking can cause a wealth of health issues including cirrhosis of the liver, high blood pressure, stroke, type 2 diabetes, weight gain, and cancer of the upper gastrointestinal tract and colon.

Foods and Nutrients to Increase

Individuals should meet the following recommendations as part of a healthy eating pattern while staying within their calorie needs.

12. **Increase vegetable and fruit intake.** Fruits and vegetables are packed with essential nutrients, many of which are under-consumed by most Americans. According to the Centers for Disease Control and Prevention (CDC), eating fruits and vegetables is associated with the reduced risk of many chronic diseases. Eating at least 2 1/2 cups of fruits and vegetables daily is associated with a reduced risk of cardiovascular disease such as heart attack and stroke. Fruits and vegetables may even help to protect against certain types of cancer. As an added bonus, most fruits and veggies are relatively low in calories. For people with type 2 diabetes, fruits and starchy vegetables should be counted into their carb count along with grains and other carb-containing foods such as beans and dairy products.

13. **Eat a variety of vegetables, especially dark-green and red and orange vegetables, as well as beans and peas.** Mom always told you to eat your spinach, but little did she know how beneficial it really is. The more color in a veggie, the more nutritional value it has. And don't forget about the dried beans and peas. Beans, peas, and legumes are excellent sources of protein, iron, zinc,

potassium, folate, and dietary fiber, and they are low in fat and calories. They are such great sources of protein and nutrients that they can be considered as both starchy vegetables and protein sources, remember to count as a carbohydrate. Consider swapping out meat a few times a week for a main dish focused on beans.

14. **Consume at least half of all grains as whole grains. Increase whole-grain intake by replacing refined grains with whole grains.** It doesn't take much to include more whole grains in your daily diet. If you get at least half of your grains from whole grains you are making a positive and beneficial change. Switch your breads to whole-wheat or whole-grain varieties, choose cereal for breakfast that is labeled "whole grain," and swap out white rice for brown rice and white pasta for whole-grain pasta. These are simple changes that can make a big difference.

Your Nutrition Solution Tidbit: Whole grains are consumed as either a single food, such as brown rice or popcorn, or as an ingredient in a food, such as buckwheat or bulgur. Other whole-grains include millet, oatmeal, quinoa, rolled oats, wild rice, whole-grain barley, whole rye, and whole wheat. It's nice to know that even popcorn is a whole grain and can be healthy if you don't top it with loads of butter and salt! Look for the whole-grain ingredient in the product to be first or second on the ingredients list.

15. **Increase intake of fat-free or low-fat milk and milk products such as milk, yogurt, cheese, or fortified soy**

beverages. Milk and milk products provide calcium, vitamin D, and potassium to our diet. This food group is essential for good bone health and is also linked to a reduced risk of cardiovascular disease and type 2 diabetes, as well as lower blood pressure in adults.

16. **Choose a variety of protein foods, which include seafood, lean meat and poultry, eggs, beans and peas, soy products, and unsalted nuts and seeds.** In addition to providing protein, these foods also supply plenty of B vitamins, including niacin, thiamin, riboflavin, and B6, as well as vitamin E, iron, zinc, and magnesium to our daily diets. The key is to consume a variety of these foods for your best nutritional intake.

17. **Increase the amount and variety of seafood consumed by choosing seafood in place of some meat and poultry.** Seafood includes fish such as salmon, tuna, trout, and tilapia, and shellfish such as shrimp, lobster, crab, and oysters. Seafood is a much healthier option as a protein source due to the type of fat it contains, which is the "good" or healthy fat. Fish and shellfish contribute many nutrients, most important of which are the omega-3 fatty acids eicosapentaenoic acid (EPA) and docosahexaenoic acid (DHA). The American Heart Association recommends consuming about 8 ounces of seafood (especially fatty fish) per week to provide enough EPA and DHA to help lower the risk of cardiovascular disease.

18. **Replace protein foods that are higher in solid fats with choices that are lower in solid fats and calories and/or are sources of oils.** The fats found in meat, poultry, and egg yolks are considered solid fats, or the "bad" fats, whereas the fats found in seafood, nuts, and seeds are considered oils, or the "good" fats. The key is

to choose lean forms of meat and poultry to decrease the amount of solid fats, and to increase your consumption of seafood, beans, soy products, nuts, and seeds as a protein source.

19. **Use oils to replace solid fats where possible.** Fats are not considered a food group but they are emphasized in the Dietary Guidelines because they supply essential fatty acids and vitamin E to our diets. Replacing some of the saturated fats with unsaturated fats can help to lower both total cholesterol and low-density lipoprotein (LDL), or the "bad" cholesterol. Unsaturated fats such as oils can be found naturally in some foods, such as olives, nuts, avocados, and seafood. Some oils are extracted from plants, such as canola, olive, corn, safflower, soybean, and sunflower oils. The key is to get more oils and fewer solid fats; also keep in mind that whether fats are healthy or unhealthy, they are all a concentrated source of calories, so use them all in moderation.

20. **Choose foods that provide more potassium, dietary fiber, calcium, and vitamin D, which are nutrients of concern in American diets. These foods include vegetables, fruits, whole grains, and milk and milk products.** All of these nutrients are emphasized in the Dietary Guidelines because, on average, most Americans do not consume enough of them.

Building Healthy Eating Patterns

21. **Select an eating pattern that meets your nutrient needs over time at an appropriate calorie level.** There are plenty of healthy eating patterns out there that

apply most of the recommendations from the Dietary Guidelines we have discussed. The USDA Food Patterns, the DASH Eating Plan (Dietary Approaches to Stop Hypertension), and the Mediterranean diet are just a few. Individuals are able to adopt these healthy eating plans to suit their personal, health, and cultural preferences.

Your Nutrition Solution Tidbit: Several studies cited in *Diabetes Care* and *Diabetes Spectrum* have revealed that diabetics who follow a Mediterranean style-eating plan lowered their A1Cs, as well as improved their cholesterol, triglycerides, and blood pressure.

22. **Account for all foods and beverages consumed and assess how they fit within a total healthy eating pattern.** Just about all foods and beverages can somehow fit into a healthy eating pattern, and that includes an eating plan for people with type 2 diabetes. The key is to first add all of the food and nutrients you need and then to fit in some of the others where possible.

23. **Follow food safety recommendations when preparing and eating foods to reduce the risk of foodborne illnesses.** Always follow safety recommendations when storing and preparing foods. Foodborne illness affects more than 76 million individuals in the United States yearly, which leads to 325,000 hospitalizations and 5,000 deaths. Keep you and your family safe by cleaning your hands, food contact surfaces, vegetables, and fruits. Separate raw, cooked, and ready-to-eat foods while shopping, storing, and preparing foods. Be sure to

cook foods to a safe temperature and refrigerate perishable foods promptly. Prevent cross-contamination by using different cutting boards, utensils, and dishes for raw and cooked meats. In addition, avoid foods that pose a high risk of foodborne illness such as unpasteurized milk, cheeses, and juices; raw or undercooked animal foods such as seafood, beef, poultry, pork, and eggs; and raw sprouts.

Source: USDA Center for Nutrition Policy and Promotion, Dietary Guidelines for Americans, www.cnpp.usda.gov/DGAs2010-PolicyDocument.htm

4. Eat Smaller Meals More Often

A good way to structure your diabetic meal plan is to eat five or six smaller meals throughout the day instead of just a few large ones. Everyone should eat this way, but it is particularly beneficial for people with type 2 diabetes. Smaller, more frequent meals generally help to keep blood glucose levels lower, resulting in smaller glucose responses and requiring less insulin. This can help improve glucose control and keep it on more of an even keel. In addition, eating smaller meals can help to control hunger, cravings, and calorie intake, increase your energy levels, and, as an added bonus, help with weight loss. It also gives you more opportunities during the day to fit in healthy foods such as fruits, vegetables, and whole grains. It is important to space your smaller meals at regular intervals throughout the day, about every three hours or so. Time them according to your waking and sleeping schedule, and keep in mind that eating too often or going too long without eating can both wreak havoc on your blood sugar levels.

Once you know approximately what your total carbohydrate intake for the day should be, you can begin planning your meals and snacks. In general, most experts recommend about 45 to 60 grams of carbs at meals and around 15 to 30 grams of carbs for snacks in between meals. Think of snacks as more of a mini-meal than a snack and try to include at least two different food groups. Be careful of late-night snacks. You don't want to eat anything too heavy in carbs too close to bedtime as you may wake up with an elevated blood sugar. However, if you have problems with nighttime hypoglycemia, you may need to adjust that. You will need to test your blood sugar and work with your RDN and/or CDE to see what schedule works best for you.

Your Nutrition Solution Tidbit: Depending on what you eat and how much, your blood sugar will begin to rise 30 to 60 minutes after eating, and it usually peaks at about one and a half to two hours after the meal. This is important to know for blood-sugar monitoring. Taking your blood sugar too soon after a meal can result in false results. The American Diabetes Association recommends (for adults) a general blood sugar target before meals of 70 to 130 mg/dL; one to two hours after beginning a meal it should be less than 180 mg/dL. Not everyone will need to monitor their blood sugar levels, but testing can provide you with feedback on how well you are managing your diabetes meal plan. You should speak with your doctor about the need for daily testing and a plan of when you need to test.

The following are snack ideas with around 15 to 30 grams of carbohydrates. Just as with meals it is always a good idea to add protein, healthy fat, and fiber to the mix when you can. In addition, just as you do with meals, make sure to pay close attention to your portion sizes and use measuring devices if needed. Don't forget that you need to add snacks to your overall carb count as well as your total calories for the day.

- 5 whole-wheat crackers + 1 piece of reduced-fat string cheese
- 2 whole-grain rice cakes + 1 Tbsp. peanut butter
- 1/3 cup hummus + 1 cup raw veggies for dipping
- 3 cups light popcorn
- 1/2 turkey sandwich in whole-wheat bread
- 1/4 cup low-fat cottage cheese + 1/2 cup canned fruit (in its own juice)
- 1/2 cup tuna salad (made with low-fat mayo) + 4 whole-wheat crackers
- 1 small piece of fruit + 15 almonds
- 6 oz. light yogurt + 3/4 cup berries
- 1 medium banana + 1 Tbsp. peanut butter
- 1 small apple + 1 Tbsp. peanut butter
- 1 whole-grain English muffin + 1 Tbsp. almond butter
- 1 hardboiled egg + 3/4 cup whole-grain cereal + 1/2 cup fat-free milk

5. Exercise Regularly

Exercise is a lifestyle habit that plays an extremely important role in managing your diabetes, your weight, and your overall health. Everyone should exercise as part of a healthy lifestyle, but for people with type 2 diabetes the stakes are even higher. Physical activity is right up there with your meal plan and medication. Exercise doesn't mean hours at the gym; it means anything that helps to get your body moving. The goal is to get active and stay active on a regular basis with a good exercise plan. Aside from specific exercise time, merely being more active in your daily routine can be helpful.

For people with type 2 diabetes exercise helps to:

- Lower overall blood sugar levels and improve A1C levels
- Maintain and/or reduce your body weight
- Keep your heart healthy by lowering both your resting heart rate and your blood pressure
- Lower "bad" cholesterol (LDL) and increase the "good" cholesterol (HDL)
- Lower triglyceride levels
- Make your body more sensitive to insulin so it can work more efficiently
- Possibly reduce your need for medication and/or insulin
- Increase circulation of the blood, especially to your extremities
- Reduce the physical and mental implications of stress and depression
- Increase your energy levels
- Facilitate better sleep
- Improve your balance and joint flexibility
- Make you feel better overall, both physically and mentally
- Decrease your risk for many other health conditions, those related to type 2 diabetes and those that are not.

Blood Glucose and Exercise

During exercise, insulin sensitivity is increased so that your cells can use glucose for energy during and also after activity. In addition, when your muscles contract during exercise and physical activity, it stimulates another mechanism separate from the action of insulin that allows your cells to absorb glucose and use it for energy, whether insulin is available or not. This is the reason exercise can help lower blood glucose short term (usually for a good 24 hours). When you exercise consistently it can help to lower your A1C as well. Always check with your healthcare provider before starting an exercise program.

The effect exercise will have on your blood sugar depends on several factors, such as how long you exercise, what type of exercise you do, and what you eat beforehand. You will need to discover and become familiar with how your body responds to exercise. Testing your blood sugar before, during, and after exercise will help you see how your body reacts to certain activities, which in turn will help you manage your blood sugar better during exercise and avoid spikes and lows.

Hypoglycemia, or low blood sugar, can occur after exercise—even 24 hours later—and you must be ready to treat it. Symptoms of hypoglycemia include shakiness, lightheadedness, weakness, confusion, fatigue, hunger, or anxiety, headaches, and breaking out into a clammy sweat. Most people with type 2 diabetes won't have a problem with this unless they use insulin or have poor blood glucose management to begin with. If you do experience low blood sugar during exercise, simply eat something with at least 15 to 20 grams of carbs that is fast-acting, such as a sports drink, juice, or a regular soft drink. Wait for about 15 minutes and check your blood sugar. Repeat this until your blood sugar is back to normal. If low blood sugar during exercise occurs regularly, speak with your doctor, RDN, and/or CDE about adjusting your meal plan, medication, and/or insulin. If you experience low blood sugar hours after exercising, eat a carb-containing snack to get your blood sugar back up to normal levels.

Follow these general guidelines for blood sugar levels and exercise:

- If your blood sugar is lower than 100 mg/dl, eat a small carb-containing snack before you begin your workout.

- If your blood sugar is between 100 and 250 mg/dL you are probably good to go. This is a safe pre-exercise level for most people with type 2 diabetes.

- If your blood sugar is 250 mg/dL or higher, use caution. Your best bet, if you are able, is to test your urine for ketones, which is a substance made when your body breaks down fat for energy. Too many ketones are an indication that your body doesn't have enough insulin to do its job and control blood sugar. Exercising at that point could cause serious complications. If you are not sure whether it is safe to exercise, contact your doctor.

- If your blood sugar is over 300 mg/dL, it is probably too high for you to safely exercise. Postpone your workout until your blood sugar levels drop to a safe range.

Getting Motivated and Sticking to It

With all of the benefits right in front of you, it is pretty hard to say no to exercise! For some it will still take a bit of motivation to get started and even more to stick to it. Here are a few tips to help you do just that:

- Set small, specific, attainable goals for yourself. Once you reach a goal, set a new one. The idea is to keep moving ahead.

- Schedule your daily exercise on your weekly calendar the way you would do anything else in your week, and stick to it.

- Use visual cues to remind and motivate yourself. Stick a note on the 'fridge or your computer, and put your workout shoes by the door.

- Get a workout buddy and exercise together.

Guidelines for Getting Started

Whether you have never exercised or are an avid exerciser, you need to do it safely. It is always a good idea to speak with your doctor first about what is safe for you and your individual situation. It is important to be aware of a few guidelines and warnings before you get started. Here are a few of them:

- Aim for 30 minutes of moderate to vigorous aerobic activity at least five days per week for a total of 150 minutes per week.

- Aim for strength training at least twice a week in addition to your aerobic exercise.

- If you have never exercised before, start slow and work your way up. Start with five to 10 minutes a day and work up from there. In time your fitness will improve and you will be able to do more for a longer period of time.

- For consistency, spread your physical activity out during the week so that you are able to exercise most days. Don't go more than two days without exercising.

- If you can't find the time for a block of 30 minutes, split your exercise up into three 10-minute increments throughout your day.

- Don't just rely on exercise for physical activity; also work more activity into your everyday life. Use the stairs, clean the house, walk the dog, wash the car— they all add up.

- The best time to eat is about 30 minutes before you exercise. You don't need an entire meal; a snack made up of at least 30 grams of carbs and some protein will do, such as half of a whole-grain bagel with peanut butter, or a banana and a handful of nuts.

- Test your blood sugar before your workout to ensure it is at a safe level for exercising.

- It is best to work out at the same time each day to help with blood sugar control.

- To be on the safe side, wear identification that states you have diabetes.

- Drink plenty of water before, during, and after exercise.

- If you have any recurring, exercise-related pain in your legs, feet, or other extremities, as well as any blisters or sores on your feet, report it to your doctor right away.

Your Nutrition Solution Tidbit: Make sure you are exercising hard enough to make a difference but not so hard that physical activity becomes too difficult. *Moderate* intensity means you can talk, but not sing, during your activity. *Vigorous* activity means you can't say more than a few words without having to stop to take a few breaths.

The Best Types of Activities

There are so many fun ways to exercise. The key is to choose something that suits you and that you enjoy doing. This will help you stay motivated and stick with it. No matter what you choose, always warm up for at least five minutes before starting your exercise and cool down for five minutes afterward. The best type of exercise program combines both aerobic activity and strength training. Aerobic exercise helps your body to better utilize insulin. It strengthens your heart, relieves stress, improves circulation, and lowers blood pressure—just to name a few benefits. Doing different types of aerobic exercise during your week helps to keep exercise more interesting and works out different parts of your body.

Examples of aerobic exercise include:

- Brisk walking
- Swimming or water aerobics
- Dancing
- Biking/spinning
- Jogging/running
- Stair climbing
- Low-impact aerobics
- Rowing
- Cross-country skiing
- Tennis
- Cardio machines such as a cross-trainer or elliptical machine

Strength training and resistance training make your body more sensitive to insulin, can help to lower blood glucose, maintain and build muscle and strengthen bones. The more muscle you have, the higher your metabolism, or the more calories you burn all the time, and not just when exercising.

This type of exercise includes weight machines, free weights, resistance bands, and exercises that use your own body weight, such as lunges, squats, and push-ups.

Stretching, flexibility, and balance exercises are another form of exercise to consider adding to your plan. This type of exercise includes basic stretches, yoga, pilates, and Tai Chi. Stretching and flexibility can help to stretch out joints and prevent stiffness. Gentle stretching for five to 10 minutes before and after exercise is great for warm-up and cool down and helps prevent injury. This can be great for relieving stress as well. Balance exercises are beneficial for people of any age, but especially for those who are aging and starting to lose a little balance. These types of exercise can help you stay steady on your feet and reduce the risk of falling and getting injured. Examples include walking backward or sideways, standing on one leg at a time, and standing from a sitting position. Exercises that strengthen your leg muscles and your lower core muscles are also good for balance. If your balance isn't great, make sure to have someone spot you as you do these exercises.

Your Nutrition Solution Tidbit: Using a pedometer to monitor how many steps you take a day can be a great way to get started with physical activity or as an addition to your exercise plan. An article in the *Harvard Health Letter* reports that a summary of 26 different studies found that people who use pedometers actually increase their activity by almost 30 percent.[2] Having a goal of 10,000 steps a day (about five miles) is important. You don't have to reach that goal at the beginning, but work your way up to it. Even taking a short walk in the morning and after meals can significantly improve 24-hour blood glucose control.

chapter 4

10 foods to avoid and 10 foods to include for type 2 diabetes

Choosing the right foods is a large part of managing type 2 diabetes. For some people with type 2 diabetes it is the sole treatment. Contrary to popular belief, there really are no foods that are totally off-limits for people with type 2 diabetes. Even though there are "good" foods and "bad" foods to consider with any healthy diet, no food is inherently evil—if you indulge only on rare occasions and watch your portion size closely. That said, many foods and beverages are *not* considered the best choices because they may wreak havoc on blood sugar. That doesn't necessarily mean they are "bad" or unhealthy foods (though some are), but that they are just not the best choices for people with type 2 diabetes. Luckily there are some good choices that may do the opposite and help you to control blood sugar. In this chapter I will discuss some of these foods and also provide a guide to sugar substitutes.

10 Common Culprits

Although people with type 2 diabetes are not truly banned from eating any certain food, there are definitely foods you want to steer clear of because they can easily spike blood sugar levels and increase the risk for diabetic complications. This list is just a sampling; as a person with type 2 diabetes you need to become a detective and investigate the foods and beverages you consume and find out if and how they can best fit into your daily meal plan.

1. **Candy and other sweet treats.** We all experience that sweet tooth from time to time, but as a person with type 2 diabetes you need to satisfy from turning to candy and other sweet treats to satisfy that need. High-sugar foods such as candy, cookies, donuts, cake, syrup, and soft drinks are known as "empty calories," foods that provide plenty of calories but little or no nutritional value. Most importantly they can wreak havoc on your blood sugar levels and your weight loss efforts. Save these sweets for special occasions, and remember to include them in your carbohydrate counts and meal plan when you do eat them. Learn to satisfy your sweet tooth another way, with high-quality carbs that contain nutrients and/or fiber such as fresh fruit, low-fat fruit yogurt, or fat-free chocolate milk. When eating a piece of fruit try to pair it with a protein choice such as peanut butter, low-fat cheese, or nuts to minimize the impact on your blood sugar. If you can't shake that sweet

tooth try sucking on a piece of sugar-free hard candy or chewing some sugar-free gum or eat a controlled amount of an allowed food and count it into your meal plan.

2. **Fruit juices.** If a fruit juice is 100-percent juice, it isn't necessarily a "bad" food. Juices like these can offer a lot more nutritional benefit than soft drinks and other sugary drinks, but for people with type 2 diabetes, juice can cause sharp spikes in blood sugar because of its concentrated source of fruit sugar and lack of fiber. A better option is whole fruit that contains more nutritional value and is rich in fiber. For breakfast, skip the glass of juice and opt for the fiber-packed whole fruit counterpart and you will be starting your day with much better blood sugar control. Whole fruit will also fill you up more and aid in weight loss.

3. **Dried fruits.** For the average person, dried fruits such as raisins, prunes, and dried apricots are not "bad" foods, but for people with type 2 diabetes they may cause a problem. They can definitely be better than eating a cookie or a candy bar, but they still can spike blood sugar quite suddenly. Dried fruits are very concentrated sources of sugar; yes, it is natural sugar rather than added sugar, but nonetheless they can increase blood sugar, and, as we have learned, the body doesn't distinguish between the two types of sugar. Sticking to whole fruit is a better option here as well.

4. **Refined grains and starches.** Refined grains and foods made with mainly white flour such as white bread, English muffins, bagels, white rice, and white pasta act much the same way as sugar in the body, and just sugar-rich foods do, starches make controlling blood sugar much more difficult and should be avoided by people with type 2 diabetes—and everyone else for that

matter. A much better option is whole grains such as whole-wheat bread, oatmeal, brown or wild rice, whole-wheat pasta, barley, quinoa, and whole-grain couscous because they contain loads of fiber that help slow down the absorption of sugar into the bloodstream. Even whole grains have an impact on blood sugar, but at a much slower rate, so be sure to watch your portion sizes and include them in your carb counts at each meal and snack.

5. **High-fructose corn syrup.** Although all sugars will spike blood sugar, high-fructose corn syrup (HFCS) is one to watch because it is included in so many foods and has some very negative health implications. HFCS has been linked to higher calorie intake, weight gain, and the increase of insulin resistance and triglycerides. HFCS represents more than 40 percent of the caloric sweeteners that are added to foods and beverages, and is the only caloric sweetener added to soft drinks in the United States. There is no way of knowing how much HFCS is in a food or beverage, but you can read the ingredient list on the food label to give you a clue. If HFCS is one of the first ingredients listed, it is safe to assume that the product contains quite a bit. Your best option is to check labels and avoid foods and beverages that contain *any* amount of HFCS. Avoiding highly processed foods and sticking more with fresh whole foods can help you to avoid HFCS. Common foods that contain HFCS are regular soft drinks, syrups, breakfast cereals, fruit juices, popsicles, fruit-flavored yogurts, ketchup, BBQ sauces, canned and jarred pasta sauces, canned soup, and canned fruits (if in syrup).

6. **Whole-fat dairy products.** Dairy products are a great source of nutrition, adding calcium, vitamin D, and

potassium as well as other essential nutrients to your daily diet. The problem occurs when you consume whole-fat dairy products. Because dairy products are an animal food, the fat they contain is saturated fat, which can raise LDL cholesterol and promote inflammation throughout the body. Studies have shown that these saturated fats can worsen insulin resistance as well, which is the last thing a person with type 2 diabetes needs. This doesn't mean you have to go dairy-free though! Fill your fridge with the fat-free and/or low-fat counterparts of these foods (fat-free milk, low-fat cheese, low-fat yogurt, and so on). This quick swap will not only help you manage your diabetes, but it will also decrease your risk of serious health conditions related to a high intake of the "bad" fats, such as heart disease and stroke. And as an added bonus, less fat means fewer calories, which is good news for individuals trying to lose weight. Dairy products are an important food group that you want to continue including in your daily meal plan.

7. **Smoothies.** Ordering a fruit smoothie when you are out and about may seem like a healthier option at the drive-through window, but beware! These beverages with real fruit can pack an unhealthy punch of calories, sugar, and carbohydrates. They may say "fat-free," but the sugar they contain will not be blood-sugar friendly. It is important to remember that liquid calories count the same as solid food. Your best option is to make your own smoothies at home. There are plenty of recipes you can find online that are diabetes-friendly; this way you will know exactly what you are drinking and how it will affect your blood sugar. This goes along with planning ahead: If you know you are going to be out and about and will need a snack, then plan ahead and

bring it with you so that you are not tempted to stop somewhere for a food or beverage that will do more harm than good.

8. **Coffee drinks.** A simple cup of coffee with fat-free milk and a sugar substitute or sugar-free flavored creamer is not a problem, but once you hit your favorite coffee house some of the choices can become a bit dangerous for a person with type 2 diabetes. Lattes, cappuccinos, espressos, frappuccinos, and iced coffee drinks can have 50 grams or more of carbohydrates and pack in plenty of sugar and calories. So beware and do a little research on your choices before you order. Many establishments offer "light" versions, but ask about nutritional facts before you order. "Light" doesn't always mean what we think it does. Choose coffee beverages that contain fat-free milk and a sugar substitute to lighten it up and make it more diabetes-friendly.

Your Nutrition Solution Tidbit: Some studies have shown that caffeine may reduce insulin sensitivity and can result in a small rise in blood sugar levels.[1] If you are having a tough time managing your blood sugar levels, switch to decaffeinated coffee for a week or two and see if your levels improve. If they do, then stick with decaf coffee and watch your caffeine intake from other beverages as well.

9. **Flavored waters.** Flavored water may seem harmless and so convenient when you are thirsty, but the hidden sugar it may contain isn't worth the price. It seems surprising that water would end up on the "avoid" list, but many flavored, bottled waters can be loaded with carbs,

sugar, and calories. With these types of beverages the label can get tricky too. They tend to add more than one serving to the label. So for example, although it may be a 20-ounce bottle that you will drink in one sitting, the label may state the bottle contains *two* servings, so the nutritional information would only be for half of the bottle. Your best option is to flavor your own bottle of water. You can use fresh lemon juice or even squeeze juice from a lime or orange for flavoring. If you need something a bit easier there are plenty of products on the market that are meant to flavor water. Look for the ones that are sugar free and contain no calories or carbs.

10. **Fast food.** Fast food can be detrimental to anyone's diet, but because people with type 2 diabetes are at such a higher risk for health conditions such as heart disease, it can be a double whammy. Most fast-food meals contain loads of calories, sodium, cholesterol, and saturated fats; they are also carb heavy. Fried foods soak up tons of oil, leading to tons of extra calories. If you choose something breaded, such as a breaded chicken sandwich, you are consuming carbs from the bun *and* from the breading. Of course, all of us are busy, and eating on the run is sometimes the only option. If you find yourself in this situation the key is to make healthier choices and not let yourself be tempted by the foods you should not have. Stay away from "supersizing" and take a look at an item's nutritional information, which all fast-food places must now disclose, before you order. Remember that you will need to fit the meal into your day's overall carb and calorie count to stay on track. Again, your best option is to always carry food with you that you know for sure will easily fit into your diet and won't mess with your blood sugar.

10 Potential Helpers

Just as some foods are known culprits for increasing blood sugar, other foods can be helpful in keeping blood sugar levels under control. That doesn't mean that one food will work magic for you, but adding these foods to a healthy meal plan can make controlling blood sugar easier for most. Many types of good foods can help, but I'm going to discuss the top 10.

1. **Black beans.** When it comes to beans or legumes, black beans are at the top of the list as a good source of magnesium, which is a glucose-regulating mineral. People with type 2 diabetes are often found to be low in this mineral, so adding black beans to your diet can be a great way to ensure you are getting enough. All beans are a winning combination of high-quality carbs, lean protein, and soluble fiber that helps to stabilize your blood sugar levels and keep hunger in check. Beans are also inexpensive, versatile, and fat-free. You can add beans to chili, casseroles, soups, salads, tacos, and burritos. Other great bean varieties are chickpeas, lentils, kidney beans, soybeans, navy beans, and pinto beans. When using canned beans rinse them thoroughly to lower the sodium content.

2. **Almonds.** Unsalted almonds provide a healthy low-carb option that contains a mix of monounsaturated fats, fiber, magnesium, and other essential nutrients such as folate, vitamin E, and potassium. Magnesium is an essential nutrient for many functions, including regulating blood glucose. Studies have shown that including plenty of almonds in your meal plan can improve insulin sensitivity and lower LDL (bad) cholesterol.[2] For those with normal blood sugar, regular consumption of nuts in general is linked to a lower risk of type

2 diabetes and heart disease. You can include nuts in your meal plan by adding them to breakfast cereal, stir-frys, salads, brown rice, and yogurt. Other great varieties of nuts are pecans, walnuts, pistachios, Brazil nuts, and cashews. Opt for the unsalted versions, and remember that even though nuts are a healthy food, just a small amount can add up in calories, so watch your portion sizes.

3. **Spinach.** Spinach is chock-full of vitamin K, vitamin A, folate, magnesium, iron, B vitamins, calcium, potassium, vitamin C, antioxidants, fiber, and a host of other goodies. It has been found to have both anti-inflammatory and anti-cancer properties. It truly is one of the super foods, and for a person with type 2 diabetes the good news is that it has an extremely low glycemic index so it will not affect blood sugar very much. Because of its low glycemic index, low carbohydrate content, and low calorie content, you can basically eat all you want. All dark-green leafy vegetables are an excellent and protective addition to your meal plan. You can eat spinach cooked or raw and can add it to soups, salads, sandwiches, lasagna, and omelets, or just eat it as a side dish. Other great greens are Swiss chard, kale, romaine lettuce, arugula, and beet greens.

4. **Salmon.** Salmon and other fatty fish such as lake trout, sardines, herring, albacore tuna, and mackerel are a great source of lean, high-quality protein, and contain no saturated fat. The type of fat they do provide is heart-healthy omega-3 fatty acid in the form of EPA (eicosapentaenoic acid) and DHA (docosahexaenoic acid). These two omega-3 fatty acids in fatty fish are known to reduce the risk for diabetes as well as improve how the body effectively uses insulin. Omega-3

fatty acids are full of protective benefits against heart disease, arthritis, and eye problems, just to name a few. Try to include at least 7 ounces of fatty fish in your diet each week. Enjoy salmon and other varieties of fish grilled, broiled, or baked.

5. **Ground flaxseed.** Ground flaxseed is rich in omega-3 fatty acids, in particular linolenic acid (ALA). They also are rich in fiber, antioxidants, and lignans. Lignans are known to improve blood sugar levels in people with type 2 diabetes. Ground flaxseed is much better absorbed than its whole counterpart. You can add 1 to 2 Tbsp. of ground flaxseed per day to your meal plan, but don't go over that. Flaxseed is usually not recommended during pregnancy. Add ground flaxseed to smoothies, non-fat yogurt, hot cereal, mashed potatoes, and baked goods.

6. **Oatmeal.** Oatmeal has always been touted as a heart-healthy food because of its cholesterol-lowering properties, and regularly consuming whole-grains is associated with a reduced risk of type 2 diabetes, heart disease, and high blood pressure. Oatmeal is a natural whole grain loaded with soluble fiber that can help slow the absorption of glucose from the food in our stomach and help control blood sugar levels. Whole grains such as oatmeal offer a steadier source of energy than refined grains and can also help with weight loss. Be careful of the type of oatmeal you choose, though. Instant oatmeal can sometimes be high in sugar so check the food label.

7. **Avocados.** Avocado is a fruit rich in monounsaturated fats, one of the healthiest fats around. They are also a good source of fiber, potassium, vitamins C and K, folate, and B6. According to The Harvard School of Public Health, tudies have shown that a diet high in

monounsaturated fat and low in refined carbs may help to improve insulin sensitivity. Monounsaturated fats also improve heart health, which is especially important for people with type 2 diabetes who are at an increased risk for heart disease and stroke. Add sliced avocado to sandwiches or salads, use them to make a healthy guacamole dip, or use guacamole on baked potatoes or grilled chicken breasts.

8. **Egg whites.** Egg whites are another healthy choice for people with type 2 diabetes and can help balance your meal plan. Egg whites are rich in high-quality lean protein and they have little to no fat and few calories. This part of the egg makes a great alternative to the yolk, the part of the egg that contains the fat and cholesterol. For people with type 2 diabetes, egg whites make a great low-calorie, high-protein option. The best part is that you can swap the egg whites for the whole egg in just about any recipe. This is not to say that whole eggs are unhealthy, but many people with type 2 diabetics deal with high cholesterol issues, and because the yolk contains all of the cholesterol in an egg, egg whites can make a great alternative. You don't even need to fully avoid whole eggs, just limit them and use egg whites more often. For example, when scrambling eggs use one whole egg and two egg whites, or make egg salad with one whole hard-boiled egg and the whites of a second.

9. **Sweet potatoes.** Sweet potatoes are packed with fiber, vitamin A, beta carotene (a powerful antioxidant), vitamin C, and potassium. What is interesting about sweet potatoes is that they may have the ability to actually improve blood sugar control, even in people with type 2 diabetes. These potatoes contain fiber and have a fairly low glycemic index, which can definitely help

with blood sugar control. However, it is believed that these two things are not what help with blood sugar control the most. Rather, it is because sweet potatoes may increase adiponectin in people with type 2 diabetes. Adiponectin is a protein hormone produced by the body's fat cells that acts as a modifier of insulin metabolism. It seems that people who have poorly regulated insulin metabolism and insulin sensitivity tend to have lower levels of adiponectin, and people with no problems when it comes to insulin metabolism have higher levels. Though more research needs to be done in this area, outcomes are looking positive. And that is good news for those who love sweet potatoes. You can bake sweet potatoes in the oven or slice them up, sprinkle them with olive oil, and bake them for sweet potato "fries."

10. **Berries.** Berries include a whole host of fruits like strawberries, black berries, blueberries, cranberries, and raspberries. These tiny fruits pack a big punch, contributing loads of fiber, antioxidants, folate, vitamin C, B vitamins, and much more. Berries are some of the best sources for antioxidants, which can help to reduce inflammation, prevent and manage arthritis, slow age-related memory loss, reduce the risk of cataracts and other eyesight problems, and reduce the risk for some cancers, heart disease, and type 2 diabetes. Blackberries are particularly high in fiber, which can help to manage type 2 diabetes. Blueberries contain two antioxidant compounds that have anti-diabetic properties and can help to improve insulin sensitivity. You can use berries on salads, in cereals, in smoothies, on yogurt, or just as a snack.

A Guide to Sugar Substitutes

When you have people with type 2 diabetes, satisfying that sweet tooth is not always easy. Including sweets in your meal plan takes careful planning and is only recommended on special occasions. One option is to try foods and drinks with sugar substitutes, also referred to as artificial sweeteners, which are synthetic sugar that may be derived from naturally occurring substances such as herbs or even sugar itself. These artificial sweeteners are many times sweeter than regular sugar, so only a small amount is needed for taste.

Sugar substitutes are broken up into two categories: nutritive (they provide the body with calories and affect blood sugar) and nonnutritive (they provide little to no calories and will not affect blood sugar). Nonnutritive sweeteners or sugar substitutes can be beneficial for people with type 2 diabetes as well as for weight loss, but the use of them is a personal preference. Sugar substitutes are in no way a magic aid for weight loss or for automatic blood sugar control, and if used should only be consumed in moderation. If you are unsure about adding them to your diabetic meal plan, speak with your doctor.

A lot of controversy surrounds sugar substitutes and their safety. We will break it all down here and give you a summary of what is available and what experts have to say. Sugar substitutes are currently regulated and approved for sale by the U.S. Food and Drug Administration (FDA) as food additives or GRAS (generally recognized as safe) products. In addition, the FDA has established an AI (Adequate Intake), the maximum daily amount considered safe to consume, for each approved artificial sweetener. The FDA's approval process is rigorous and reviews many factors, including determination of probable intake, cumulative effect from all uses, and toxicology studies in animals.

Sugar Substitutes Available

There are currently six products determined to be safe and approved for use in the United States by the FDA: acesulfame K, aspartame, neotame, saccharin, sucralose, and stevia. All have different functional properties and tastes.

- **Acesulfame K (sold as Sweet One, Sunett).** This sweetener has no caloric value and is 200 times sweeter than table sugar. It is heat stable and blends well with other sweeteners so it can be used for cooking and baking.

- **Aspartame (sold as NutraSweet, Equal).** This sweetener has been around for more than 20 years. It contains 4 calories per gram and is 160 to 220 times sweeter than table sugar. It is not heat stable so it's not recommended for cooking or baking. Because it contains phenylalanine, people with phenylketonuria (PKU), a rare genetic disorder, should not use aspartame.

- **Neotame (made by NutraSweet).** This sweetener is 7,000 to 13,000 times sweeter than table sugar. It is heat stable and has a milder aftertaste than some of the other artificial sweeteners. Even though this product is similar to aspartame, it does not carry a warning for individuals with PKU because the metabolism of it reduces the availability of phenylalanine.

- **Saccharin (sold as Sweet 'N Low, Sweet Twin, Sugar Twin).** This sweetener has no caloric value and is 200 to 700 times sweeter than table sugar. This product is heat stable. Although people have been concerned about the safety of saccharin since the 1970s, according to the Beverage Institute for Health and Wellness, studies have determined that saccharin is safe for human consumption.

- ⋈ **Sucralose (sold as Splenda).** This sweetener is 600 times sweeter than table sugar and is made directly from sugar but is not considered a natural product. This product is heat stable so it can be used in cooking and baking.

- ⋈ **Stevia (sold as Truvia, PureVia, Steviva, Sun Crystals, A Sweet Leaf).** This sweetener is 200 times sweeter than table sugar. It is extracted from the leaves of the stevia plant, which is native to South America. The highly purified extract of stevia is called Rebaudioside A (or Reb A). It is heat stable so it can be used in a variety of foods. Only the Reb A form of stevia is recognized as GRAS by the FDA, so look for that form when choosing a stevia product.

Your Nutrition Solution Tidbit: If you find nutritive sweeteners on a food ingredient list, keep in mind that food or beverage will affect your blood sugar. These include sweeteners such as glucose, fructose, white or table sugar, lactose, galactose, brown sugar, dextrin, maple syrup, maltose, raw sugar, corn sweetener, dextrose, honey, molasses, high-fructose corn syrup, invert sugar, agave nectar, and corn syrup.

A Word About Sugar Alcohols

I briefly mentioned sugar alcohols earlier in this book, but it is important to go a little more in depth. Sugar alcohols, also referred to as polyols, are also considered sugar substitutes and have been used in food products for many years to help decrease the intake of carbohydrates. These types of sugar substitutes are manufactured carbs for use in food products, and they also occur naturally in certain fruits and vegetables. They can be used alone in food products but are usually used in combination with other nonnutritive sweeteners. Though they carry the word "alcohol" in the name, they do not contain ethanol, which is found in alcoholic beverages. Sugar alcohols are very low in calories and convert to glucose much more slowly than regular sugar. On average, they contain about 2 calories per gram, which is half the calories of other sweeteners. When you calculate the carb content of food that contains sugar alcohols, you can subtract half of the sugar alcohol grams from the total carbohydrates.

Examples of sugar alcohols are:

- Sorbitol
- Xylitol
- Lactitol
- Mannitol
- Erythritol (does not cause laxative side effects like other sugar alcohols sometimes do)
- Hydrogenated starch hydrolysates
- Isomalt

Most of these sweeteners are used to sweeten sugar-free gum and candies as well as other dietetic food products, manufactured baked goods, toothpaste, and fruit spreads. Sugar alcohols help to keep foods moist and add volume to products. Consuming too many sugar alcohols at one time can cause cramping, gas, and diarrhea in some people.

Your Nutrition Solution Tidbit: Just because a food is labeled "Sugar Free" or "No Sugar Added" does not always mean it automatically contains little to no calories or carbohydrates. The food can contain carbohydrates in another form, such as, flour or even contain fat and protein—and, therefore, calories. These products can still affect your blood sugar. Always make sure to read the label before assuming a food is a "free" food, and has no carbs and will not affect your meal plan and blood sugars.

What the Experts Have to Say

It is the position of the **Academy of Nutrition and Dietetics** that "consumers can safely enjoy a range of nutritive sweeteners and nonnutritive sweeteners (NNS) when consumed within an eating plan that is guided by current federal nutrition recommendations, such as the Dietary Guidelines for Americans and the Dietary Reference Intakes (RDI), as well as the individual health goals and personal preference."

The **American Diabetes Association** states, "Sugar alcohols and nonnutritive sweeteners are safe when consumed within the daily intake levels established by the Food and Drug Administration."

The **American Heart Association** states, "Replacing sugary foods and drinks with sugar-free options containing nonnutritive sweeteners is one way to limit calories and achieve or maintain a healthy weight. Also, when used to replace foods and drinks with added sugars, it can help people with diabetes manage blood glucose levels. For example, swapping a full-calorie soda with a diet soda is one way of not increasing blood glucose levels while satisfying a sweet tooth."

The **American Academy of Family Physicians** states, "Consumers can be assured that the use of these intense sweeteners poses no health risk. Probably the most widespread nutrition problem facing Americans today is the over-consumption of calories, leading to overweight and obesity. These substitute sweeteners, when used appropriately, can help reduce calorie intake."

chapter 5

menu planning and shopping guide

Now that you have learned how to plan your meals and eat more healthily for type 2 diabetes, it is time to get out there and put your plan into action by preparing menus and going grocery shopping. There will be times when sticking to a meal plan will get a bit tricky, so I will provide some tips to help get you through those times. Properly navigating the grocery store and mastering food labels will be two tools in your arsenal that will get you through all types of food situations and make you feel more confident in your efforts to manage your type 2 diabetes.

Menu Planning Tips

As a person with type 2 diabetes food is something you must pay close attention to. Eating more healthily, managing carbohydrates, timing meals, and controlling portions are all crucial to managing your blood sugar. I've discussed all of these previously in the book, but here are a few more tips to help you more easily plan your daily menus and be prepared for special circumstances.

- The best way to make managing type 2 diabetes less difficult is to plan ahead! Write out your menus for the week so that you can plan meals that appropriately time and portion out your carb intake. This will make managing your blood glucose much easier. You need to ask yourself where and when you will be eating in the next week and how much time you will have to cook. The more prepared you are, the less likely you will be to eat out, eat on the run, or grab something you shouldn't, all of which can spell trouble for your blood sugar. Once your menus are planned you can create your shopping list. This will help you to buy only what is on your list and not stray to foods you should avoid.

- Plan for eating small meals more frequently instead of two to three large ones. You will need to plan not only meals but also healthy snacks or mini-meals that will help keep your blood sugar stable throughout the day. Don't forget to plan for meals or snacks that need to be taken to work or school.

- Don't meal plan separately for you and the family. Buy a few recipe books or look online for some healthy, easy, and tasty recipes that the whole family will enjoy.

- When planning your menus add the foods that can benefit blood-sugar management, such as beans, nuts, green leafy vegetables, salmon, and some of the other foods I mentioned in Chapter 4. Look up some new recipes that incorporate some of these foods and try something new!

ℵ   Be creative and come up with some yummy substitutions in your menus for the foods you need to limit so that you don't feel deprived. (More on this in the next section.)

> **Your Nutrition Solution Tidbit:** If you are not one to sit down and write things out, grab your phone and find an app for that! There are plenty out there that make planning your shopping list easy and fun.

Swap It Out

A diagnosis of type 2 diabetes can bring many changes, especially in the foods you eat. It can be hard to give up some of your favorite foods that you were used to eating on a regular basis. But the good news is that there is no need to feel deprived if you learn to make some smart and simple swaps that can lower calories, carbs, sugars, and fats. The following list will get you started, but as you get used to your new eating style you will be able to figure out all kinds of yummy and healthy swaps!

Instead of:	Try:
Cream pie	Yogurt, non-fat, light, in the same flavor
Ice cream	Light frozen yogurt or sugar-free ice cream

Ice cream sundae	Parfait with non-fat, light vanilla yogurt, berries, and low-fat granola
Milkshake	Milkshake made with frozen yogurt or sugar-free ice cream and a favorite fruit
Chocolate cake	Chocolate pudding, fat-free, sugar-free, with light whipped topping
Cinnamon roll	Toasted whole-grain English muffin sprinkled with a touch of cinnamon
Apple pie	Fresh apple, sliced, with non-fat, light yogurt for dipping
Fast-food French fries	Frozen fries or freshly cut potato (white or sweet potato), oven-baked
Potato chips and dip	Homemade guacamole and raw veggies
Pizza	Homemade whole-wheat pita bread, no-sugar pizza sauce, part-skim mozzarella cheese, veggies, and turkey sausage
Beef burger	Turkey burger or portabella mushroom, grilled; use a lettuce wrap or a 100-calorie, thin, whole-grain sandwich bagel instead of a bun; add lettuce, tomato, and other favorite toppings, with mashed avocado instead of mayo

Dining Out

Eating out is not an excuse to break the rules when you have type 2 diabetes. You still need to follow your carbohydrate meal plan and be diligent about your food choices, but you can still have an enjoyable meal. Here are a few tips to help you out:

- Plan ahead and make a mental note of portion sizes and how many carbs you will be allowed at the meal.

- Do not "save up" your carbs for your restaurant meal. Eat as you normally would throughout the day and at the meal.

- If you are going to eat at a different time than you normally would, reorganize the timing of your meals and snacks for the day to avoid any blood sugar issues.

- Obtain a copy of the restaurant's nutritional information before you go so that you can have a good idea of what to order when you get there. Most restaurants have nutrition information listed on their Websites.

- Don't be afraid to ask questions or ask to have your food prepared a certain way. They are there to serve *you!*

- Most restaurant portion sizes are much larger than what you will need. Ask for a doggie bag when you order your meal and put half the entrée away before you begin to eat. That way you won't be tempted to over-indulge and eat the whole meal.

⋊ Order dressings and sauces on the side so that you have more control of what you are putting on your food.

⋊ Ask for substitutions. If your meal comes with French fries ask for a salad or fresh fruit bowl instead or even a plain baked potato.

⋊ Be careful of the bread they bring the table. If it doesn't fit into the carb count for your meal, stay away. If you want the bread, make the necessary changes to your main meal.

⋊ Choose meats or fish that are not breaded and are broiled, baked, or grilled instead.

Feeling Under the Weather

When you are feeling a bit under the weather it may not be possible to stick to your normal meal plan. In addition, when you are sick and your body is under stress it releases certain hormones to help your body deal with the stress, and these hormones can raise blood sugar and affect the utilization of insulin. So your blood sugar becomes harder to control, not only because you are not able to eat as you normally would, but also because of what your body is going through. For these reasons it is important to take precautions when you are ill. The best way to prevent a minor illness from becoming a major problem is to have a plan of action already in place. Having a plan in place will make you feel more at ease because you will know how to handle it and have needed supplies on hand. The last thing you want to be doing when you are not feeling well is worrying about what to eat. Ask your doctor to help you work out an action plan for sick days.

Your action plan might include some of the following:

❧ Check your blood glucose more often, and check your urine ketones (speak with your doctor or CDE if you don't have a meter to check this). Record your readings and contact your doctor if your blood sugar or ketones reach abnormal levels.

❧ Continue to take your medication, whether it is insulin or oral medication. If you take medication and/or insulin, chances are that when you are ill you may need to adjust them, so it is a good idea to contact your doctor, especially if you are unable to keep your oral meds down.

❧ Make sure your sick-day plan includes a substitute meal plan, one that is better suited for when you are not feeling well. Try to consume your normal amount of calories, especially the carbs. The meal plan can include carb foods that are gentle on your stomach such as soups, crackers, dry toast, applesauce, gelatin, and tea.

❧ If you are not able to handle solid foods, your plan will need to contain liquids and liquid-type foods that contain carbs (not sugar-free) such as juice, frozen juice bars, sherbet, regular pudding, creamed soup, regular gelatin, broth, sports drinks, and fruit yogurt. Consume these liquids in small amounts and aim for about 50 grams of carbs every three to four hours.

❧ Sip plenty of water throughout the day when you are sick to avoid becoming dehydrated. You can try other sugar-free beverages as well, but stick to those that are caffeine-free.

⋈ Even with a plan in place, call your doctor if these problems arise:

   ⋈ You have been sick with a fever for a couple days and it doesn't seem to be getting better.

   ⋈ You have been vomiting and/or had diarrhea for more than six hours.

   ⋈ You have a change in mental status and feel fuzzy or confused.

   ⋈ You have high to moderate levels of ketones in your urine.

   ⋈ Your glucose levels are higher than 240 mg/dL even though you have taken the extra insulin and/or medication your sick-day plan calls for.

   ⋈ You have any symptoms that may indicate dehydration or something more serious.

Your Nutrition Solution Tidbit: Before you take any over-the-counter medications for a cold or other ailment, call your doctor to ensure it is safe for you to take.

Celebrating the Holidays

Holidays are always fun, but they tend to center or lots and lots of food! This can be difficult for people who deal with managing type 2 diabetes on a daily basis. But that does not mean you too can't enjoy the holiday festivities. It just takes a little extra planning and preparation. It will be well worth it for both your health and your holiday enjoyment.

⋈ The key is to plan in advance so that you can lessen your stress and anxiety concerning what to eat, how much to eat, and when to eat. This will allow you to more fully enjoy your holiday and keep your blood sugar levels in check.

- If you take insulin or an oral medication that lowers blood glucose levels, don't wait to eat if you are eating away from home. You may need to grab a healthy carb snack at your normal mealtime to keep from going too low.

- Don't forget to continue physical activity. This can help you manage calories and your blood sugar levels.

- Try healthier versions of your favorite holiday dishes. For example, add a bit less sugar to your pie, try baking with a sugar substitute, or add lower-fat ingredients to your favorite casserole.

- If you are not hosting the holiday and are going to friends' or families' homes, bring a diabetic-friendly dish to share. No one will know it is diabetic-friendly, and *you* will know for sure that you have something you can rely on to eat that won't cause too many problems for you.

- Do not avoid meals or snacks during the day to save up for a big holiday meal later! This can cause all types of problems for you and your blood sugar. Continue to eat throughout the day as you normally would and continue with your carb counting. You can eat just a bit lighter in calories if you know you will be eating more than usual at the big meal, but do your best to stay consistent throughout the day.

- You can try just about everything at the holiday meal; just take smaller portions so you don't overdo it.

Navigating the Supermarket

Consuming a diet that will help you manage your type 2 diabetes starts long before you sit down to eat—it starts at the supermarket. When you go to buy food for your home you need to be armed with a well-thought-out meal plan, a weekly menu, and a grocery list. Even with all of that in your arsenal, wheeling your cart down each isle at the grocery store can be overwhelming. Make sure you have plenty of time when you shop so that you can shop wisely, and eat a healthy meal or snack *before* you go shopping. Going shopping hungry can be your worst enemy!

You can also check your grocery store's Website before heading out. Many of the larger chains allow you to create an online shopping list, and many also offer guidelines and meal ideas for people with type 2 diabetes. In addition, many large chains now have a dietitian on the premises, so if you get stuck on a food or have questions, don't be afraid to ask! That is what they are there for.

Grocery stores can be tough, with all of the foods available staring you in the face at every turn. That's why your number-one weapon is a well-organized and well-thought-out grocery list that follows the menu plan you developed for the week. Here are a few tips to arm yourself with the next time you go grocery shopping so that you'll be able to fill your cart with the healthiest foods from each aisle.

The Fruits and Vegetables Section

The first section you will come to in most grocery stores is the produce section, full of fresh fruits and vegetables. This section of the grocery store is probably the largest and the one you should spend most of your time in. Fruits and vegetables make great healthy snacks and should be included with meals and snacks as often as possible. Most vegetables are low in carbs, so if you are going to go overboard with any food, make it one of these. Fruit can even be a great substitute for dessert or when you have a sweet tooth. Here are some tips for navigating this section of the grocery store.

- Look for produce with the most color. The more colorful a vegetable is, the more nutrients it contains. There are plenty to choose from: broccoli, red peppers, spinach, carrots, sweet potatoes, and red grapes, just to name a few. Even white veggies such as onions and cauliflower contain loads of beneficial nutrients too.

- Choose a variety of fruits and vegetables each time you shop. Variety is the spice of life, and the more variety you choose, the more nutritional value you will get. Be adventurous and try something new every week. You never know what you'll find that you really like. Always remember to add them to your carb count at meals and snacks.

- Buy fruits and vegetables that are in season and, better yet, locally grown. Organic options are always a great idea but can also be costly.

- Pre-cut fruits and vegetables are a great idea for the busy person.

- Buy fresh, frozen, or canned (in 100-percent juice; make sure there is no syrup) versions so that you always have something on hand.

- Keep in mind that dried fruits such as apricots, raisins, and prunes can be much higher in carbs per serving than fresh fruit. Check labels for serving size and carbs they contain.

- When buying fresh buy only what you need so that you can eat it up before it goes bad.

✯ Nuts and seeds are often found in this section, and should be a part of your grocery list. They add healthy fat, fiber, and other nutritional value to your meal plan.

The Dairy Section

The dairy section usually lines the perimeter of the grocery store. Even though it is usually labeled "the dairy case" it is filled with all types of foods—some in the dairy food group and some not—such as milk and milk alternatives, such as soy milk, yogurts, cheeses, sour cream, cream cheese, eggs, puddings, butter and margarine, and dips. Here are some tips for navigating this section of the grocery store.

✯ Stick to the low-fat and fat-free versions throughout the dairy case to lower your intake of unhealthy saturated fats.

✯ If using margarines or spreads, check the label for the words "partially hydrogenated" in the list of ingredients. These are the unhealthy trans fats and should be avoided at all costs! Many margarine spreads are now made without trans fats.

✯ Choose yogurts that are fat free or low fat as well as "light" or sugar free. Greek yogurt is a good option because it provides more protein than regular yogurts.

✯ Although eggs are considered a protein choice, you can find them, as well as egg-white substitutes, in this section. Egg-white substitutes are a good alternative for whole eggs and a great way to lower your fat and cholesterol intake.

The Meats and Seafood Section

This area of the grocery store, again in the "fresh" perimeter of the store, includes fresh meats, seafood, fish, and the deli section. Meats, especially red meats, can contain high amounts of unhealthy saturated fats and calories, so the goal here is to choose more lean meats and fish to help decrease your risk for heart disease. Here are some tips for navigating this section of the grocery store.

- Choose lean-meat choices such as skinless white meat poultry, fish (wild caught), pork loin, pork tenderloin, top sirloin steak, eye of round roast or steak, sirloin tip side steak, top round roast and steak, bottom round roast and steak, flank steak, chuck shoulder pot roast and steak, extra-lean ground beef (at least 90-percent lean), and extra-lean ground turkey. Cuts of meat are considered lean if they include the words "round" or "loin."

- For luncheon meats choose lean turkey, roast beef, lean ham, or chicken breast, and stay away from high-fat meats such bologna and salami. Keep an eye on sodium content as well.

- Opt for fewer red meats and more poultry and fish.

Your Nutrition Solution Tidbit: The American Heart Association recommends at least two servings of fish per week. Salmon is a great choice because it is widely available, affordable, not too "fishy," and a good source of omega-3 fatty acids.

The Breads/Cereal/Rice/Pasta Sections

As you get into the center aisles of the grocery store you will encounter fewer fresh foods and more packaged and processed foods such as breads, cereals, rice, and pasta. This section offers you a great way to get your daily whole-grain and dietary fiber intake as well as other essential nutrients—if you make the right choices. This is also the "carb" section, so tread lightly here and be sure to read food labels closely. Here are some tips for navigating this section of the grocery store.

⊠ Avoid refined foods such as white breads, regular pasta, white rice, and sugary cereals.

⊠ Choose oatmeal, as it is not only a whole grain and high in fiber but also a benefit to those with type 2 diabetes. Regular oatmeal is a better choice than instant because it is less processed, but even instant oatmeal is a whole grain and a good choice if you pay attention to the sugar and carb content.

⊠ When choosing dry cereals, choose varieties that state "whole grain" and aim for at least 4 grams of fiber per serving. Read the label for sugar content and stick to those with the lowest.

⊠ Choose whole-wheat or whole-grain breads, cereals, and pasta, and other high-fiber, whole-grain foods such as brown and wild rice. Try alternating your usual whole grains for something different, such as bulgur, quinoa, barley, and whole-grain couscous, to keep your meals interesting.

⊠ Reading food labels is key in all sections, but especially in this one. You will need to read labels to ensure you are choosing foods that are truly whole grains and have the fiber content you expect.

The Canned Food Sections

The canned food sections include fruits, vegetables, tuna, beans, soups, and more. Keeping a variety of healthy canned goods on hand can ensure you always have something to reach for in a pinch. Even though they're not fresh, these foods can still add to your required daily servings of certain foods groups. Canned foods can be just as nutritious if you make the right choices. Here are some tips for navigating this section of the grocery store.

- Choose fruit that is canned in water or its own natural juices to keep sugar and carb content down. Stay away from any that state "in syrup."
- Choose vegetables without added salt.
- Avoid buying frozen or canned vegetables that contain sodium or added fats such as sauces or butter. No need to ruin a good thing!
- Choose tuna that is packed in water as opposed to oil.
- Choose low-fat soups and try to stick with the broth-based soups that contain loads of vegetables.
- Choose beans such as black, kidney, lentils, garbanzo, and navy, with no added salt. Add them to soups, casseroles, whole-wheat pastas, and salads as an extra protein, nutrient, and fiber boost. Rinse canned beans to remove as much sodium as possible.

The Oils, Condiments, and Dressings Section

This can be a dangerous section as it is filled with fats and sodium. But it just takes making some good choices to get through this aisle in a healthy manner. Here are some tips for navigating this section of the grocery store.

- ⋊ Choose healthier oils such as extra virgin olive oil and canola oil, and use them sparingly. A little bit can go a long way and can pack in a lot of calories.

- ⋊ Keep in mind that ketchup, salsa, and other condiments may contain sugar. Look for low-sugar versions or choose brands with the lowest amount of sugar and carb per serving.

- ⋊ Choose salad dressings that are oil-based and reduced-fat. Compare labels to choose those lower in sodium and sugar. Your best choice for salad dressing is a little extra virgin olive oil with apple cider vinegar.

- ⋊ Try replacing regular mayonnaise with a reduced-fat or fat-free version, or try pre-packaged guacamole instead, for something a bit more nutritious.

- ⋊ Grab a can of fat-free cooking spray to use in sautéing and baking to save some calories.

Your Nutrition Solution Tidbit: When choosing olive oil, opt for extra virgin, which is the purest form of olive oil with the lowest acidity. This oil is great for dressings, drizzling on vegetables, or brushing on breads. If you plan to cook with the oil it is best to go with virgin or light olive oil as they are better suited for heating. Always check dates, because oils have a limited shelf life, and choose a bottle from the back of the shelf, because light tends to destroy the oil and its properties. Store it in a cool, dark, dry place once you get home.

The Frozen Foods Section

The frozen foods section includes a large variety of foods: vegetables, fruits, pizza, frozen entrees, breakfast foods such as pancakes and waffles, specialty items, breads, juices, ice cream...and the list goes on. Frozen fruits and vegetables are a convenient way to always have produce on hand, especially during the winter months. Frozen foods can make cooking more convenient, and, with the right choices, a bit more diabetic-friendly. Here are some tips for navigating this section of the grocery store.

- Be sure to read labels in the freezer section so that you always choose healthier varieties. For example, if you are choosing frozen breakfast foods, opt for whole-grain waffles.

- Choose vegetables that do not include sauce and butter. Many frozen vegetables come in ready-to-steam bags, which makes adding vegetables to meals even easier. Having frozen vegetables on hand means you can always throw extra vegetables in soups, casseroles, pasta, and stews, or just add them as a side dish.

- Choose frozen fruit without added sugar. Frozen fruits are great for making smoothies or adding to your whole-grain waffles for breakfast or yogurt as a snack.

- If choosing frozen meals/entrées you will need to read the nutrition facts panel. These meals are fine on occasion when you don't have time to cook, but don't rely on them regularly. In general, look for meals that include vegetables, whole grains, and lean meat, fish, or poultry. Skip those that are sky-high in carbs and those that include cream sauces, gravies, or fried foods, as well as those that contain more than 600 mg of sodium. Don't assume these meals are healthy without first checking the label.

⋈ Instead of ice cream, choose low-fat frozen yogurt or other sugar-free treats to eat on occasion.

Using Food Labels to Help Manage Type 2 Diabetes

It is time to become a label reader so that you can determine, without guessing, whether a food is healthy and whether it will fit within the guidelines of your diabetic meal plan. The food label is regulated by the FDA and is full of information including the Nutrition Facts Panel, Nutrient Content Claims, and Health Claims. Food labels are meant to be used by the consumer to compare foods and make better choices. They are especially helpful for type 2 diabetics who use carb counting as a way to plan meals.

The Nutrition Facts Panel

The "Nutrition Facts Panel" provides consumers with information about nutrients people are most concerned about. This panel is the rectangular box on the back or side of food and beverage packaging that contains all of the nutritional information. The Nutrition Facts Panel was mandated under the Nutrition Labeling and Education Act (NLEA) of 1990 and is based on recommendations from the Food and Drug Administration (FDA) and the U.S. Department of Agriculture (USDA).

Nutrition Facts

Serving Size 1 cup (228g)
Servings Per Container about 2

Amount Per Serving

Calories 250   Calories from Fat 110

	% Daily Value*
Total Fat 12g	18%
Saturated Fat 3g	15%
Trans Fat 3g	
Cholesterol 30mg	10%
Sodium 470mg	20%
Total Carbohydrate 31g	10%
Dietary Fiber 0g	0%
Sugars 5g	
Proteins 5g	
Vitamin A	4%
Vitamin C	2%
Calcium	20%
Iron	4%

* Percent Daily Values are based on a 2,000 calorie diet. Your Daily Values may be higher or lower depending on your calorie needs:

	Calories:	2,000	2,500
Total Fat	Less than	65g	80g
Saturated Fat	Less than	20g	25g
Cholesterol	Less than	300mg	300mg
Sodium	Less than	2,400mg	2,400mg
Total Carbohydrate		300g	375g
Dietary Fiber		25g	30g

For educational purposes only. This label does not meet the labeling requirements described in 21 CFR 101.9.

You can use the Nutrition Facts Panel to your advantage by following a few simple tips.

Size It Up

One of the first parts of the panel is the serving size, which is usually expressed in weight, volume, or number of units. Take a close look at the serving size and the servings per container. Ask yourself:

- How many calories are in a single serving?
- How many calories are in the entire package?
- How many servings do I plan to eat?
- Will my diabetic portion size be different?

Remember that *all* of the information on the panel pertains to one single serving size. If you plan on eating two servings, you need to double all of the information: calories, nutrients such as fat, and %DV (percent daily value). When comparing calories and nutrients on the same food but between brands, make sure you check to see if the serving size is the same.

> **Your Nutrition Solution Tidbit:** Many packages, including beverages, contain more than one serving. Don't fall into the trap of assuming there is only one serving in a package and consuming the whole package before you read the label first. That can add up to a lot more carbs, calories, and fat than you planned for.

Focus on Calories

Next on the panel are calories and calories from fat. This area is important for determining whether a food is appropriate for someone with type 2 diabetes, especially if you are trying to lose weight. We know high-fat foods can mean more calories, and, in time, weight gain.

Whether you are focusing on losing weight or maintaining a healthy weight, keep in mind that even if a food is fat-free, that doesn't make it calorie-free! Check to see how many total calories the food contains and how many of those calories come from fat. For example, if a food has 300 calories per serving and 150 of those calories come from fat, then half of the calories in a single serving come from a fat source. Consider how the calories per serving will fit into your total calorie goals for the day. The key is to keep your calories in check as you manage your weight. Keep in mind that if you eat and drink more calories than you burn, you *will* gain weight.

In general, you can use the following quick guide to gauge the calories in a single product (based on a 2,000-calorie diet), but when it comes to body weight what really matters is the total calories you consume in a day and not what is in a single food.

LOW in calories = 40 calories per serving

Moderate in calories = 100 calories per serving

HIGH in calories = 400 calories or more per serving

Total Carbohydrates

The total carbs listed on the label is a very important number to people with type 2 diabetes! Total carbohydrates includes complex carbs (starches), sugars, sugar alcohols, and fiber. Because all types of carbs affect blood sugar it is necessary to use *total* carbs when carb counting, not just grams of sugar. Because fiber does not affect blood sugar the way other carbs do, you can subtract the grams of fiber from the total carbs listed when carb counting. In addition, if sugar alcohols are listed, you can subtract half of those grams from the total carbs.

Limit These Nutrients

The nutrients listed first on the panel are the ones most Americans generally consume enough of—or too much of—in their diet. These are nutrients to limit, and they include total fat, saturated fat, trans fat, cholesterol, and sodium. It is important to know how much total fat is in a serving of a food as well as what type of fat it is. Saturated and trans fats are the ones you want to limit because we know they increase the risk for heart disease. The fats you want to include are monounsaturated and polyunsaturated fats, as they are healthy fats.

> **Your Nutrition Solution Tidbit:** The American Diabetes Association recommends, in general, choosing foods with less than 400 mg of sodium per serving. But keep in mind your daily total allowance as well.

Get Enough of These Nutrients

The nutrients listed next on the panel are nutrients that most Americans *don't* get enough of in their diet. These include dietary fiber, vitamin A, vitamin C, calcium, and iron. Eating enough of these nutrients can help improve health and reduce the risk of some health conditions and diseases. Eating a diet high in fiber promotes better blood sugar control and can also help with weight loss and maintenance.

Figuring Out Percent Daily Value

If you are not sure whether a food is high or low in beneficial nutrients, the percent daily value (%DV) tool on the panel can help you with that. First read the footnote on the bottom of the panel, which tells you that %DVs are based on a 2,000-calorie diet. This statement must appear on all food labels. This part of the food panel is the same on all labels, and does not change from product to product, as does the rest of the information. This information is recommended dietary advice for all Americans and is not specific to the food product. Remember that for a lot of people with type 2 diabetes, especially those who already have heart issues, the recommended value for sodium is 1,500 mg.

*Percent Daily Values are based on a 2,000 calorie diet. Your Daily Values may be higher or lower depending on your calorie needs:

	Calories:	2,000	2,500
Total Fat	Less than	65g	80g
Saturated Fat	Less than	20g	25g
Cholesterol	Less than	300mg	300mg
Sodium	Less than	2,400mg	2,400mg
Total Carbohydrate		300g	375g
Dietary Fiber		25g	30g

For educational purposes only. This label does not meet the labeling requirements described in 21 CFR 101.9.

As you learned from the footnote on the panel, the recommendations for total fat, saturated fat, carbohydrates, and fiber are all based on a 2,000-calorie diet, so if you eat less than or more than that calorie level, you need to adjust the recommended dietary advice to fit your individual needs. However, cholesterol and sodium recommendations are the same no matter what calorie level you are consuming. The following chart shows you how the percent daily value needs to be adjusted according to calorie level.

Adjusted Percent Daily Values for Specific Calorie Levels	
Calories	Adjusted %DV
1,200	60 percent
1,400	70 percent
1,600	80 percent
2,000	100 percent
2,200	110 percent
2,500	125 percent
2,800	140 percent
3,200	160 percent

Putting %DV to Use For You

Now that we know what the daily values are we can use then to determine percent daily value (%DV), which will help you decide whether a food is high or low in a nutrient and, ultimately, if it is a smart food to choose. The %DV is listed to the right of most of the nutrients on the top part of the panel.

To help you decide quickly, use this guide:

5% DV or less is considered low for that nutrient

20% DV or more is considered high for that nutrient

Get enough of these nutrients *(The goal is to stay above 100% DV for each of these for the entire day)*: fiber, vitamin A, vitamin C, calcium, and iron.

Limit these nutrients *(The goal is to stay below 100% DV for each of these for the entire day)*: Total fat*, saturated fat, cholesterol, and sodium.

Stick to mostly polyunsaturated and monounsaturated fats, which are healthier fats.

You can use %DV not only to figure out if a food is high or low in a nutrient but also to compare products. You can easily compare one product or brand to a similar product to make the better choice. Just make sure when you compare that the serving sizes are similar. They are kept generally consistent for similar types of foods to make comparing them easier for the consumer. You can also use %DV to help you make dietary trade-offs with other foods throughout the day. This allows you to eat all of your favorite foods on occasion, and fit them into a healthy diet. For instance, when one of your favorite foods is high in fat you can balance it with foods that are low in fat at other times of the day. But pay attention to how much you eat of that favorite food so that the total amount of fat for your day stays below the 100% DV.

One more way to use %DV is to help you distinguish one dietary claim from another, such as "light" versus "reduced fat." All you need to do is compare the %DVs for total fat in each of the foods to determine which one is higher or lower in that nutrient. This way there is no need to memorize all of the definitions that go along with those claims.

Additional Nutrient Information

The label also provides %DVs for a few vitamins and minerals, including vitamins A and C, calcium, and iron. You may see more on some labels but you will at minimum always see these four nutrients. Read the %DV given so that you know how much one serving of a food contributes to the total amount you need per day.

The daily values used for these four nutrients are as follows:

- Vitamin A: 5,000 IU
- Vitamin C: 60 mg
- Calcium: 1,000 mg
- Iron: 18 mg*

For certain populations some of these numbers may be higher or lower; these are general values.

For example, if calcium is listed as 25% DV, then one serving of that food will provide you with a quarter of what you need for the day, or 250 mg.

Always check labels, and don't make assumptions. Just because yogurt is supposed to be a good calcium source doesn't mean every yogurt has the same amount of calcium. Before you buy, compare brands and choose the ones that have the most calcium and protein and the lowest sugar and fat content. Labels are on food products for the consumer, so use them!

Your Nutrition Solution Tidbit: %DVs for trans fats, sugar, and protein have yet not been established; however, you can still compare total amounts between brands to pick the better product.

Putting It All Together

Once you have checked out all parts of the panel you need to ask yourself if this particular food is a smart choice. Does it fit into a healthy diet, into your weight management plan, and, most importantly, into your diabetic meal plan? Ask these questions:

- Is one serving size enough for me, or do I need to double or triple the carbs, calories, fat, and other nutrients on the label?
- Are the calories per serving low, moderate, or high? How many calories will be in the actual amount I eat?
- Are the nutrients that I need to limit low, and are the nutrients I need more of high?
- Is this food too high in fat, especially saturated and trans fats?
- What are the total grams of carbs, and how will they fit into my planned meal?
- Does this food contain too many carbs for my needs? Are these carbs mostly sugar?
- Will this food provide me with some needed fiber?
- Have I compared the label on this product to those of other brands to ensure I am getting the most bang for my buck? Should I look for an alternative?

How you answer these questions will depend on your calorie intake, whether you are trying to lose, maintain, or gain weight, whether you might have specific nutritional needs, and how well your blood glucose is being controlled. The bottom line is that food labels enable you to compare foods based on key ingredients and therefore make better choices for your type 2 diabetes meal plan. Food labels allow you to include your favorite foods occasionally, even if they are not always the smartest choices. Use the nutrition facts panel to make your food choices easier and healthier!

Nutrient content Claims on Food Labels

Even if you don't have time to read each and every food label, something known as "nutrient cntent claims" can help you to quickly find foods that meet your specific needs and goals. By FDA definition, a nutrient content claim on a food product directly or by implication characterizes the level of a nutrient in a food. Examples of this characterization are "low fat," "fat free," "high in fiber," and "reduced sugar." Each and every claim used on food packaging has a specific, regulated definition. These are a few of the more popular ones that are used on food labels:

- **Reduced** or **Less:** At least 25% less total fat, saturated fat, sugar, sodium, or cholesterol, or 25% fewer calories than the regular product. This might not necessarily mean the product is actually *low* in a nutrient if the regular product is quite high.

- **Light** or **Lite:** 1/3 fewer calories or no more than half the fat of the regular, higher-calorie, higher-fat version; or no more than half the sodium of the regular, higher-sodium version.

- **Good Source, Contains,** or **Provides:** Between 10 and 19 percent of the daily value for a nutrient per serving.

- **Excellent Source Of, High,** or **Rich In:** 20 percent or more of the daily value for a nutrient per serving.

- **More, Fortified, Enriched, Added, Extra,** or **Plus:** 10 percent or more of the daily value for a nutrient per serving compared to the regular product.

- **No Added Sugars:** No sugar or sugar-containing ingredient is added during processing.

- **Sugar Free:** less than 0.5 grams of sugar per serving.

- **Low Fat:** 3 grams of fat or less per serving.

- **Fat Free:** less than 0.5 grams of fat per serving.

- **Cholesterol Free:** less than 2 milligrams cholesterol and 2 grams or less of saturated fat per serving.

- **Low Sodium:** 140 mg or less of sodium per serving.

- **Sodium Free:** less than 5 milligrams of sodium per serving.

- **Low Calorie:** 40 calories or fewer per serving.

- **Calorie Free:** fewer than 5 calories per serving.

- **Lean (on meat labels):** less than 10 grams of fat per serving, with 4.5 grams or less of saturated fat and 95 milligrams of cholesterol per serving.

- **Extra Lean** (on meat labels): less than 5 grams of fat per serving, with less than 2 grams of saturated fat and 95 milligrams of cholesterol.

Health Claims on Food labels

Health claims on labels are another tool to help you make healthier choices that are individualized to you and your health issues. By FDA definition, a health claim is any statement made on the label or in the labeling of a food or dietary supplement that expressly or by implication (such as through third-party references, written statements, symbols, or vignettes) characterizes the relationship of any substance to a disease or health-related condition. Implied health claims include those statements, symbols, vignettes, or other forms of communication that suggest, within the context in which they are presented, that a relationship exists between the presence or level of a substance in the food and a disease or health-related condition.

Here are a few health claims you've probably seen:

- "Diets rich in whole-grain foods and other plant foods and low in total fat, saturated fat, and cholesterol may help reduce the risk of heart disease."

- "Low-fat diets rich in fiber-containing grain products, fruits, and vegetables may reduce the risk of some types of cancer, a disease associated with many factors."

To find all of the nutrient content claims and health claims visit the FDA at *www.fda.gov*.

Your Nutrition Solution Tidbit: Need a little more help choosing the right foods? Look for these icons on food packages:

Whole Grains Council Stamp: The 100% stamp means that *all* of the grain in the product is whole grain (at least 16 grams of whole grains per serving). The basic stamp means the product may contain some extra bran, germ, or refined flour (at least 8 grams of whole grains per serving).

Heart-Check Mark: The food product meets the nutrition requirements of the American Heart Association.

chapter 6

14-day menu guide and stocking your kitchen

By now you have a great deal of information that will help you start using nutrition as a large part of managing your type 2 diabetes. Now I'll help you put it all together by providing 14 days of menus to get you off on the right foot. You can use these menus as a starting point to help you plan your own menus according to your individual likes and dislikes. In addition, this chapter will provide you with an extensive list of all of the foods and beverages that are great to have on hand in your kitchen if you are actively managing type 2 diabetes.

14-Day Menu Guide

The following menus give you approximately 1,800 to 2,000 calories per day, so you may need to adjust portion sizes depending on your individual calorie needs. All the menus are low in "bad" fats (saturated and trans fats) and are an excellent source of "good" fats (polyunsaturated and monounsaturated as well as omega-3 fatty acids). In addition, they are a good source of high-quality protein and fiber. They consist of approximately 50 percent carbohydrates, 20 percent fats, and 30 percent protein, with the general recommendation of 45 to 60 grams of carbs at meals and 15 to 30 grams of carbs at snacks. These menus avoid the common foods that are not best for people with type 2 diabetes and include the foods that may benefit you. The format of these menus follows the recommendation of frequent and smaller meals throughout the day. A bedtime snack is provided, but that may not be appropriate for everyone, so it is important to create a menu plan with your RDN and/or CDE that will work for you. You will need to adjust the timing of your meals if, for example, you work second or third shift and go to bed at an unusual hour. Beverages are not included with these menus, except for milk. Drink plenty of water throughout your day and choose non-caloric beverages with meals.

Day 1

breakfast

1 cup steel-cut oats, cooked with water, topped with 1/2 cup fresh sliced strawberries and sprinkled with cinnamon

4 egg whites, scrambled

8 oz. fat-free milk

<u>a.m. snack</u>

1 cup low-fat cottage cheese

1/2 cup peach slices, fresh or canned in their own juice

<u>lunch</u>

Smoothie: mix together in blender 3/4 cup fresh or frozen blueberries (no sugar added); 1/2 large banana, chilled; 6 oz. light, low-fat vanilla yogurt (no sugar added); 1 Tbsp. ground flaxseed

2 multigrain rice cakes

<u>p.m. snack</u>

4 celery stalks

2 Tbsp. peanut butter

20 grapes

<u>dinner</u>

Turkey burger, grilled or broiled, with 1/2 cup avocado, pureed or cubed; 3 spinach leaves; 1/4 cup diced tomato; in 1/2 of a 6-inch whole-grain pita

2 cups salad with greens and raw veggies, topped with 2 tsp. oil and vinegar

<u>bedtime snack (if needed)</u>

1 orange

10 unsalted almonds

Day 2

breakfast

1 1/2 cups whole-grain dry cereal, low sugar, topped with 1/2 cup fresh blackberries and 8 oz. fat-free milk

2 slices Canadian bacon, heated

a.m. snack

8 whole-grain crackers

1 oz. Swiss cheese, low-fat

1 hard-boiled egg

lunch

Sandwich: 5 oz. turkey breast; 1/4 cup pureed avocado; 1/2 cup diced tomato; 2 leaves romaine lettuce; 1 oz. cheddar cheese, low-fat; in half of a 6-inch whole-grain pita

1 apple

p.m. snack

1/4 cup hummus

6 baby carrots

dinner

6 oz. skinless chicken breast, grilled or broiled, topped with 1 Tbsp. lite Teriyaki sauce

3/4 cup brown rice, cooked

1 cup broccoli, steamed

8 oz. fat-free milk

bedtime snack (if needed)

6 oz. low-fat, Greek yogurt, no sugar added, topped with 1/2 cup raspberries, fresh or frozen, and 1 Tbsp. ground flaxseed

Day 3

breakfast

2 slices whole-wheat bread, toasted, spread with 1 Tbsp. peanut butter

2 links turkey sausage

1 cup strawberries, fresh, sliced

8 oz. fat-free milk

a.m. snack

6 oz. low-fat yogurt, no sugar added

7 walnut halves

lunch

Wrap: 3 oz. skinless chicken breast, cooked; 2 oz. black beans, rinsed; 1/4 cup cheddar cheese, shredded; 1/4 cup spinach, chopped; 2 Tbsp. salsa, low-sugar; rolled into one 10-inch whole-wheat tortilla

1 orange

8 oz. fat-free milk

p.m. snack

2 graham cracker rectangles

20 grapes

<u>dinner</u>

6 oz. salmon, grilled, baked, or broiled

Pasta: 3/4 cup whole-wheat pasta, cooked, with 1 cup zucchini, steamed; 1/2 cup tomatoes, diced; 1/2 Tbsp. extra virgin olive oil

<u>bedtime snack (if needed)</u>

3/4 cup low-fat cottage cheese

1/2 cup pineapple chunks, in its own juice

Day 4

<u>breakfast</u>

2 whole-grain waffles (4-inches round), spread with 1 1/2 Tbsp. almond butter

1 1/2 cup cantaloupe

8 oz. fat-free milk

<u>a.m. snack</u>

1 cup sugar-free gelatin, any flavor, mixed with 3/4 cup blueberries

<u>lunch</u>

Tuna salad sandwich: 3 oz. tuna, light, canned in water; 1 Tbsp. low-fat mayo; 1/2 Tbsp. relish; 1/4 cup celery, diced; 2 spinach leaves; stuffed into half of a 6-inch whole-wheat pita

2 cups vegetable soup, light

<u>p.m. snack</u>
1 apple
2 multigrain rice cakes

<u>dinner</u>
6 oz. flank steak, broiled or grilled
1 medium sweet potato baked in skin, with 1/2 Tbsp. margarine, trans-fat free
10 asparagus spears, fresh, steamed
1 cup carrots, steamed
8 oz. fat-free milk

<u>bedtime snack (if needed)</u>
1 banana, spread with 1 Tbsp. peanut butter

Day 5

<u>breakfast</u>
Omelet: 4 egg whites and 1 whole egg; 1/4 cup lean ham, diced; 1/4 red bell pepper, diced; 1 oz. mozzarella cheese, part-skim
2 slices whole-wheat bread, toasted, with 1 Tbsp. margarine, trans fat-free
1 cup honeydew melon, diced

<u>a.m. snack</u>
1 apple, spread with 1 Tbsp. peanut butter

lunch

Black bean salad: 4 oz. black beans, rinsed; 1/4 cup tomatoes, diced; 1/2 cup cucumber, peeled and diced; 1/4 cup bell pepper, diced; 1/4 cup avocado, diced; 1 tsp. fresh lemon or lime juice; sprinkle of garlic powder; salt and pepper to taste

8 oz. fat-free milk

p.m. snack

1/4 cup hummus

8 crackers, whole-grain, low-salt

dinner

Stir-fry: 6 oz. shrimp, cooked; 1 cup broccoli flower clusters; 1/2 cup carrot slices; 1 cup snow pea pods; 1/4 cup water chestnuts; 2 Tbsp. soy sauce, light; 1 Tbsp. extra virgin olive oil; 1/2 cup brown rice, cooked

bedtime snack (if needed)

3/4 cottage cheese, low-fat, with 1 cup sliced strawberries

Day 6

breakfast

Smoothie: 3/4 cup fresh or frozen strawberries (no sugar added); 1/2 large banana, chilled; 6 oz. light, low-fat vanilla yogurt (no sugar added); 1 Tbsp. ground flaxseed

2 slices whole-wheat toast

1 Tbsp. margarine (trans-fat free)

a.m. snack
1 hard-boiled egg

2 rice cakes, multigrain

20 grapes, red

lunch
Wrap: 1/2 cup refried beans, fat-free, warmed; 1/4 cup cheddar cheese, low-fat, shredded; 1 Tbsp. chopped onions; 2 Tbsp. salsa, low-sugar; in one 10-inch whole-wheat tortilla

1 pear

p.m. snack
2 cups vegetable soup, low-sodium, low-fat

dinner
Pasta: 3 lean turkey meatballs; 1/2 cup pasta sauce, low-sugar; 3/4 cup spaghetti, whole-wheat, cooked; 1 Tbsp. Parmesan cheese, freshly grated

2 cups salad greens topped with fresh vegetables, with 2 tsp. oil and vinegar dressing

8 oz. fat-free milk

bedtime snack (if needed)
10 almonds, unsalted

1/2 cup cheddar cheese, low-fat, diced

8 oz. fat-free milk

Day 7

<u>breakfast</u>

1 cup steel-cut oats, cooked with water, topped with 1/2 cup fresh blueberries, sprinkled with cinnamon

2 lean turkey sausage links

8 oz. fat-free milk

<u>a.m. snack</u>

1 banana, spread with 1/2 Tbsp. almond butter

<u>lunch</u>

Sandwich: 1/2 whole-wheat pita, stuffed with 3 slices lean ham; 1 slice Swiss cheese, low-fat; 2 slices tomato; 2 spinach leaves; 1/2 tsp. mustard

1 orange

8 oz. fat-free milk

<u>p.m. snack</u>

1/4 cup hummus

3 celery stalks

1 cup red bell pepper slices

<u>dinner</u>

6 oz. pork tenderloin, baked or grilled

1 medium sweet potato, baked in skin, with 1 Tbsp. margarine, trans-fat free

1 cup broccoli, streamed

1 cup cauliflower, steamed

<u>bedtime snack (if needed)</u>
1 cup strawberries, sliced, topped with 1/4 cup whipped topping, light (no sugar added)

7 walnut halves

Day 8

<u>breakfast</u>
Breakfast sandwich: 4 egg whites, scrambled; 1 oz. low-fat Swiss cheese; 2 slices Canadian bacon, cooked; on 1 whole-wheat English muffin, toasted

1/2 pink grapefruit, sprinkled with sugar substitute

1 cup milk, fat-free

<u>a.m. snack</u>
6 oz. fruit yogurt, no-fat, sugar-free, fruited, with 1/2 cup raspberries, fresh or frozen (no sugar added), and 1 Tbsp. ground flaxseed

<u>lunch</u>
Chicken salad: 3 oz. chicken breast, chopped; 1/4 cup celery, diced; 2 Tbsp. low-fat mayo; 1/2 Tbsp. relish; in one 10-inch, whole-wheat tortilla

1 apple

8 oz. fat-free milk

<u>p.m. snack</u>
1 cup sugar-free gelatin, mixed with 1 cup peaches, fresh or canned in own juice, topped with 2 Tbsp. whipped topping, light, no sugar added; 5 pecans

<u>dinner</u>

6 oz. halibut, grilled, baked, or broiled

1 cup wild rice, cooked

10 spears asparagus, steamed

2 cups salad greens with raw veggies, with 2 tsp. oil and vinegar dressing

<u>bedtime snack (if needed)</u>

4 cups popcorn, light

1/4 cup pistachios, no shell

Day 9

<u>breakfast</u>

1 1/2 cups whole-grain dry cereal, low sugar, topped with 1/2 cup fresh blackberries

1 hard-boiled egg

8 oz. fat-free milk

<u>a.m. snack</u>

2 rice cakes, multigrain

1/2 cup cheddar cheese, low-fat, cubed

<u>lunch</u>

Salad: 3 oz. chicken breast, sliced; 3 cups romaine lettuce; 1/2 cup broccoli, raw; 1/2 cup carrots, grated; 1/2 cup cucumbers, sliced; 1/2 cup red bell peppers, sliced; 1/2 cup garbanzo beans, rinsed; 1 Tbsp. oil and vinegar dressing

Crumble 10 baked tortilla chips on top

p.m. snack

1 graham cracker rectangle with 1 Tbsp. peanut butter

8 oz. fat-free milk

dinner

6 oz. low-fat turkey kielbasa, grilled, baked, or broiled

1 Tbsp. ketchup

1 1/2 cup spaghetti squash; 1 1/2 cup zucchini, steamed; with 1 Tbsp. margarine, trans-fat free

1 cup cantaloupe, diced

bedtime snack (if needed)

3/4 cottage cheese, low-fat, with 1/2 cup pineapple, canned in its own juice

Day 10

breakfast

Smoothie: 3/4 cup fresh or frozen blueberries (no sugar added); 1/2 large banana, chilled; 6 oz. light, low-fat vanilla yogurt (no sugar added); 1 Tbsp. ground flaxseed

2 lean turkey sausage links, cooked

a.m. snack

1 whole-wheat English muffin, toasted, spread with 1/4 cup mashed avocado

lunch

Tuna salad: 3 oz. light tuna, canned in water; 1/4 cup celery, diced; 1 Tbsp. low-fat mayo; 1/2 Tbsp. relish

10 whole-grain crackers

8 baby carrots

1 medium kiwi fruit

8 oz. fat-free milk

p.m. snack

1 cup Sugar-free pudding, low-fat

1/2 banana, sliced

dinner

Tacos: 3 oz. lean ground turkey breast, cooked with taco seasoning, low-salt; 1/2 cup blacked beans, rinsed and heated; 1/4 cup cheddar cheese, low-fat, shredded; 1/2 cup tomatoes, diced; 1/4 cup black olives, sliced; 2 tortilla shells or two 6-inch, whole-grain soft tortillas

2 cups salad greens with raw veggies, with 2 tsp. oil and vinegar dressing

8 oz. fat-free milk

bedtime snack (if needed)

4 cups popcorn, light

10 almonds

Day 11

<u>breakfast</u>

Egg-white omelet: 4 egg whites; 1/4 cup chopped mushrooms; 1 Tbsp. chopped onion; 1/2 cup chopped green pepper; 1/4 cup cheddar cheese, low-fat, shredded

Directions: In a non-stick skillet, sauté veggies in a small amount of olive oil until tender. Add egg whites and cook until set. Flip omelet and cook until done. Add cheese and fold.

2 slices pumpernickel bread, toasted, with 1 Tbsp. margarine, trans-fat free

1/2 grapefruit, pink, sprinkled with sugar substitute

8 oz. fat-free milk

<u>a.m. snack</u>

1 apple spread with 1 Tbsp. peanut butter

<u>lunch</u>

Bean dip: 1/2 cup refried beans, fat-free; 1/4 cup avocado, mashed/pureed; 1 Tbsp. onion, chopped; 1/2 cup tomato, diced; 1 oz. cheddar cheese, low-fat, shredded;

Directions: Spread ingredients in small layers in a bowl

10 tortilla chips, baked, for dipping

1 pear

<u>p.m. snack</u>

6 oz. Greek yogurt, non-fat, sugar-free

5 vanilla wafer cookies, reduced-fat

<u>dinner</u>

Beef kabobs: 6 oz. sirloin steak, cubed; 3 mushrooms, sliced; 1 small onion, cut in chunks; 1/2 sweet red pepper, cut in chunks; 6 cherry tomatoes

Directions: Combine beef and vegetables in 2 Tbsp. reduced-fat Italian dressing and 2 Tbsp. light Teriyaki sauce, and let sit at least two hours, covered, in fridge. Arrange beef and veggies on two skewers, and grill or broil, rotating until beef reaches an internal temp of 145°F.

1 cup wild rice, cooked

1 medium peach, sliced

<u>bedtime snack (if needed)</u>

1 orange

10 almonds

Day 12

<u>breakfast</u>

2 whole-grain waffles, spread with 2 Tbsp. peanut butter

1 1/2 cup cantaloupe

8 oz. fat-free milk

<u>a.m. snack</u>

2 rice cakes, multigrain

1 hard-boiled egg

lunch

Veggie pita pizza: 1 (6-inch) whole-wheat pita; 1/4 cup tomato or pizza sauce, no added sugar; 1/4 cup mozzarella cheese,
part skim, shredded; 1 Tbsp. chopped onion; 1/4 cup green
pepper, chopped; 1/4 cup tomato, diced; 1/4 cup mushrooms,
chopped

Directions: Place pita on baking sheet sprayed with non-
stick cooking spray. Spread sauce on pita, and top with cheese
and vegetables. Bake at 450°F for about 8 min. or until cheese
is melted and vegetables are tender.

8 oz. fat-free milk

1 plum, fresh

p.m. snack

1 cup sugar-free pudding, low-fat

1/2 banana, sliced

dinner

6 oz. salmon, grilled, baked, or broiled

1 medium potato, baked in skin, topped with 1/4 cup
pureed avocado

1 cup broccoli, steamed

1 cup cauliflower, steamed

bedtime snack (if needed)

1 cup cottage cheese, low-fat

1/2 cup peaches, sliced, fresh, or canned in their own juice

Day 13

breakfast

2 slices pumpernickel bread, toasted, spread with 1 Tbsp.
almond butter

2 links turkey sausage

1 cup strawberries, fresh, sliced

8 oz. fat-free milk

a.m. snack

4 celery stalks with 1 Tbsp. peanut butter

20 grapes, red

lunch

Sandwich: 5 oz. turkey breast; 1/4 cup avocado, pureed; 1/4
cup diced tomato; 2 leaves romaine lettuce; 1 oz. Swiss cheese,
low-fat; in half of a 6-inch whole-grain pita

1 apple

p.m. snack

1 cup blackberries, fresh, topped with 1/4 cup whipped topping, light (no sugar added)

5 pecans

dinner

Baked, breaded chicken: 6 oz. skinless chicken breast; 1
Tbsp. Parmesan cheese, freshly grated; 1/4 cup crushed whole-
grain crackers; dash of paprika; dash of garlic powder; 1 Tbsp.
margarine, trans fat-free

Directions: In a bowl, combine cracker crumbs, Parmesan cheese, paprika, and garlic powder. Coat chicken with margarine, then roll it in crumbs. Bake in oven at about 350°F until juices run clear and chicken is thoroughly done.

1 1/2 cups butternut squash, baked, with 1 Tbsp. margarine, trans-fat free

1 cup spinach, chopped, steamed

8 oz. fat-free milk

<u>bedtime snack (if needed)</u>

1 kiwi fruit

1/2 oz. sunflower seeds, dry roasted, no added salt

Day 14

<u>breakfast</u>

Breakfast sandwich: 4 egg whites, scrambled; 1 oz. low-fat Swiss cheese; 3 slices turkey bacon, cooked; on 1 English muffin, whole-wheat, toasted

1/2 pink grapefruit, sprinkled with sugar-substitute

1 cup milk, fat-free

<u>a.m. snack</u>

6 oz. yogurt, non-fat, no added sugar, fruited

5 vanilla wafers, reduced-fat

<u>lunch</u>

Tuna salad sandwich: 3 oz. tuna, light, canned in water; 1 Tbsp. low-fat mayo; 1/2 Tbsp. relish; 1/4 cup celery, diced;

rolled into one 10-inch whole-wheat tortilla with 2 spinach leaves

2 cups vegetable soup, light

2 plums

p.m. snack

1/4 cup hummus

10 baked tortilla chips

1/2 cup red bell pepper, sliced

dinner

Sauté: 4 oz. lean ground turkey breast; 2 Tbsp. diced onion; 2 Tbsp. chopped green pepper; 1 tsp. chili powder; 1/4 cup salsa, low sugar; 1/4 cup tomato sauce, low sugar; 1/2 cup kidney beans

Directions: Brown ground turkey in saucepan with onion and pepper. Drain fat, add remaining ingredients, and bring to boil. Reduce heat to low and simmer for 20 min.

1/2 whole-wheat pita, toasted, with 1/2 Tbsp. margarine (trans-fat free) and garlic powder

8 oz. fat-free milk

bedtime snack (if needed)

1 cup sugar-free gelatin, any flavor, topped with 1/4 cup whipped topping, light, no sugar added, and 1/2 cup raspberries, fresh or frozen (no added sugar)

Your Nutrition Solution Tidbit: There are shakes on the market today made just for people with type

2 diabetes. They can be a good addition to your meal plan in a pinch or when you don't have time for a snack. They can be good to carry with you if needed. However, make sure you check out the label and add them into your carb count.

Stocking Your Kitchen

A well-stocked kitchen with plenty of healthy, diabetic-friendly foods will make life much easier. When you know you can grab a snack or a quick meal with the foods you have in your kitchen it will relieve some of your stress and anxiety about managing your type 2 diabetes. You might just find that your whole family will eat more healthily once your have your kitchen stocked the right way. The following list is just sampling of foods to get you started. There are many more you can add; just make sure they are on your safe and healthy lists.

Pantry

Whole-grain breads, pitas, and wraps

Oatmeal, regular, long-cooking

A variety of whole-grain, low-sugar dry cereals

Brown and/or wild rice

Quinoa

Whole-grain couscous

Pasta, whole-grain

Microwave popcorn, light

Whole-grain crackers

Graham crackers

Rice cakes

Baked tortilla chips

A variety of beans, canned or dried (black, navy, red, lima, lentils, chickpeas, soybeans, etc.)

Refried beans, fat-free

Nuts and seeds

A variety of canned soups, light (reduced fat, reduced sodium)

Broth, fat-free, sodium-free

A variety of canned vegetables with no salt added

A variety of canned fruit, in water or its own juice

Potatoes, sweet potatoes, and other root vegetables

Peanut butter

Nut butters such as almond butter

Canned tuna, light

Apple cider vinegar

Rice vinegar, flavored

Extra-virgin olive oil, canola oil, sunflower oil, and safflower oil

Herbs and spices

Ground flaxseed

Refrigerator

Milks including fat-free cows milk, almond milk, soymilk

Low-fat cheeses and cottage cheese

Reduced-fat sour cream and cream cheese

Non-fat, no sugar added yogurt (Greek yogurt is higher in protein)

Sugar-free pudding

Sugar-free gelatin

Low-fat mayonnaise

Margarine (trans-fat free) or a light butter made with good oils

Salad dressings, reduced-fat, low sugar

Hummus

Guacamole

Low-fat deli meats such as turkey or chicken

A variety of non-starchy fresh vegetables

A variety of fresh fruits

Note: Store meats in the refrigerator for only a few days. It is best to freeze meats and then thaw them for a day or two before using. Meats should be lean and can include extra-lean ground beef, lean cuts of beef, skinless poultry, and lean cuts of pork, fish, and other seafood.

Freezer

Frozen vegetables without sauces

Frozen fruits with no added sugar

Frozen yogurt or low-fat, sugar-free ice cream

Sherbet/sorbet

Frozen waffles, pancakes, French toast, all whole-grain

Frozen entrées (look for less than 600 mg sodium, plenty of vegetables, and whole grains)

appendix

ask the dietitian

We have covered a lot of information in this book, but there are always more questions to be answered. Here are a few questions I frequently hear that might just be something you need answered as well.

Q. Does drinking diet soft drinks and other diet beverages raise your blood sugar?

A. Diet soft drinks and other diet drinks don't directly raise your blood sugar. However—and this is highly debated—it is believed that artificial sweeteners or sugar substitutes may trick the brain into secreting insulin, and when there is no glucose or blood sugar to be metabolized it produces the craving to get some. So no, it will not physically raise your blood sugar, but it can possibly interfere with insulin production and produce cravings for more sweet foods. Again, this is debated, and not 100-percent scientifically proven. Your best bet is to drink diet soft drinks only on occasion because both regular and diet soft drinks contain phosphates that are just not good for you. Stick to healthier options and try to get to the point at which you are using diet soft drinks on occasion as a treat rather than every day.

Q. My mom has type 2 diabetes. Do I have a greater chance of getting it?

A. Type 2 diabetes does have a stronger genetic link than type 1 diabetes does, but just because your mom or other family member has it doesn't mean you will get it for sure. However, it may put you at greater risk. Lifestyle also contributes to type 2 diabetes, and we know that obesity plays a big part. Obesity tends to run in families, as do eating and exercise habits, so it is sometimes difficult to determine whether genetics or lifestyle is the bigger contributor.

Q. If I am overweight or obese will I eventually develop type 2 diabetes no matter what?

A. If you are overweight or obese, you won't *necessarily* develop type 2 diabetes, *but* your chances are going to be much greater than they would be for someone who is at a healthy weight. Not everyone who is overweight or obese has type 2 diabetes, and not everyone who has type 2 diabetes is overweight, which suggests there are other risk factors at work. Research is now finding that the majority of people diagnosed with type 2 diabetes didn't begin showing symptoms of the disease until they had been overweight or obese for a number of years. Just a moderate weight loss, a mere 10 percent of your body weight, can significantly reduce your risk of type 2 diabetes as well as high cholesterol and heart disease.

Q. What does my blood pressure have to do with my diabetes?

A. When you have diabetes you have a higher risk of high blood pressure (hypertension) because diabetes tends to damage arteries, making them a target for hardening of the arteries, or atherosclerosis. Atherosclerosis is what causes high blood pressure. If high blood pressure is not properly treated, it can lead to heart attack, stroke, heart failure, and even kidney failure. High blood pressure can also worsen many of the complications that people with type 2 diabetes deal with, including eye disease and kidney disease. Most people with type 2 diabetes will deal with high blood pressure at some point so it is imperative to have your blood pressure checked often and to be treated properly if you have been diagnosed with high blood pressure.

Q. Will my high cholesterol levels affect my type 2 diabetes?

A. People with type 2 diabetes are twice as likely to have abnormal lipid levels including cholesterol and triglycerides than people who do not have diabetes. Obesity, insulin resistance, and high levels of insulin can cause these abnormal levels. People who have low HDL ("good" cholesterol) and high LDL ("bad" cholesterol) are at an even higher risk for heart disease. People with type 2 diabetes can improve their cholesterol levels with better blood sugar control, regular exercise, a healthy diet, and weight loss. Taking cholesterol-lowering mediations may be needed if lifestyle changes don't do the job.

Q. Is having hyperglycemia or hypoglycemia the same thing as having type 2 diabetes?

A. Hyperglycemia and hypoglycemia are not the same as type 2 diabetes. They instead are possible symptoms of diabetes. *Hyperglycemia* is the medical term for high blood sugar and is usually characterized by a blood sugar level above 180 mg/dL. Hyperglycemia can happen when the body is making little to no insulin or is making enough insulin but not using it effectively. Having high blood sugar levels frequently or for long periods of time can cause serious health complications for people with type 2diabetes. Hyperglycemia can occur in type 2 diabetes from eating too many carbs or just not watching your diet, stress from illness and other stressful situations, not taking medication and/or insulin correctly, decreased activity, and/or strenuous activity. Symptoms can include increased thirst, headaches, frequent urination, weight loss, fatigue, and difficulty concentrating. *Hypoglycemia* is the medical term for low blood sugar and is usually characterized by a blood sugar level less than 70 mg/dL. Hypoglycemia can occur in people with and without type 2 diabetes and usually occurs due to not eating enough, or strenuous exercise without eating enough. It can also be a symptom of certain medical conditions or a side effect from certain medications. Symptoms can include shakiness, anxiety, sweating, confusion, headaches, sleepiness, and blurred vision. Usually eating something concentrated in sugar is enough to get blood sugar back up to normal levels.

Q. Can eating too much sugar cause diabetes?

A. The myth of eating too much sugar being the cause of type 2 diabetes is not that simple to address. Type 1 diabetes is caused by genetics and unknown factors that trigger the onset of the disease and has nothing to do with the amount of sugar you eat. We also know that type 2 diabetes can be caused by genetics and/or lifestyle factors. Some of these lifestyle factors include being obese or overweight, and a diet high in calories from any food source, including sugar, is one factor that contributes to being overweight or obese. So even though sugar itself may not directly cause type 2 diabetes, consuming too much can cause obesity, which in turn can increase the risk for the disease. The American Diabetes Association states that there may be a link between drinking sugary drinks and type 2 diabetes. Therefore the ADA does recommend limiting your intake of sugar-sweetened beverages to help prevent type 2 diabetes. These drinks, which include regular soft drinks, energy drinks, sports drinks, fruit drinks, and other sugar-containing beverages, can increase your blood glucose and provide an enormous amount of empty calories—calories that have no nutritional value attached to them. Limiting these beverages can help you to lose or manage weight as well. The bottom line is, "everything in moderation."

Q. If I have type 2 diabetes do I need to stay away from *all* sugar?

A. In the past, people with type 2 diabetes were always told to avoid any foods that included added sugar. Added sugar is just that: sugar that is added to a food versus sugar that occurs naturally in a food such as fructose in fruit and lactose in dairy products. This is no longer the recommendation. Added sugar should definitely be eaten in moderation and intake should be limited, but you can fit such foods into a healthy type 2 diabetic meal plan. If you take insulin, you need to calculate your dose based on the number of carbohydrates (including added sugars or natural sugars) in the food. If you take oral meds or manage your diabetes with diet alone you need to add these foods to your carb count. Many times foods with added sugars are not the healthiest options because they usually don't contain a whole lot of nutritional value. So even though you can fit them safely into your diet, it is best to do that occasionally and in moderation.

Q. Can type 2 diabetes turn into type 1 diabetes?

A. No, these are two different diseases. Type 1 diabetes is caused by different factors than those that cause type 2 diabetes. People with type 2 diabetes make no insulin and need to take insulin to survive. And even though some people with type 2 diabetes may need to take insulin injections as well, this does not mean that their disease has progressed or will progress to type 1 diabetes.

Q. Are there apps available for people with type 2 diabetes on my smart phone?

A. There are numerous apps available to help you more easily manage your type 2 diabetes, from grocery shopping to carb counting to monitoring your blood glucose. As with all apps out there, some are better than others, and it really depends on what you personally are looking for help with. Some are available for free and others you will need to pay for. No matter what types of apps you use, never use them as a substitute for regular visits to your doctor, dietitian, and/or CDE. Because apps are coming and going all the time, your best option is to do a little research. Ask your doctor, RDN, or CDE if they recommend any, and ask others who have type 2 diabetes what they are using and if it is working for them. It will be a personal decision in the end but it helps to have input before you decide.

notes

Chapter 1

1. Hanley, A.J., A.J. Karter, K. Williams, A. Festa, R.B. D'Agostino Jr, L.E. Wagenknecht, and S.M. Haffner. "Prediction of type 2 diabetes mellitus with alternative definitions of the metabolic syndrome: The Insulin Resistance Atherosclerosis Study." Circulation 112.24 (August 2005): 3713–3721.

Chapter 2

1. Linos, A., V. Kaklamani, E. Kaklamani, Y. Koumantaki, E. Giziaki, S. Papazoglou, and C. Mantzoros. "Dietary factors in relation to rheumatoid arthritis: A role for olive oil and cooked vegetables?" *American Journal of Clinical Nutrition* 70.6 (December 1999): 1077–1082.

2. "Vitamin D and Health." The Nutrition Source, a Website by the Harvard School of Public Health. *www.hsph.harvard.edu/nutritionsource/vitamin-d/*.

3. Larsson, S.C., and A. Wolk. "Magnesium intake and risk of type 2 diabetes: A meta-analysis." *Journal of Internal Medicine* 262.2 (August 2007): 208–214.

4. Abhimanyu, G., MD. "Insulin Resistance in the Pathogenesis of Dyslipidemia." Diabetes Care 19.4 (April 1996): 387–389.

Chapter 3

1. World Health Organization. "Draft Guideline: Sugars intake for adults and children." www.who.int/nutrition/sugars_public_consultation/en/.

2. "Counting Every Step You Take." *Harvard Health Letter*, September 2009. *www.health.harvard.edu/ newsletters/Harvard_Health_Letter/2009/September/ counting-every-step-you-take*.

Chapter 4

1. Keijzers, G.B., B.E. De Galan, C.J. Tack, and P. Smits. "Caffeine can decrease insulin sensitivity in humans." *Diabetes Care* 25.2 (2002): 364–369.

2. Jenkins, D.J., C.W. Kendall, A. Marchie, A.R. Josse, T.H. Nguyen, D.A. Faulkner, K.G. Lapsley, and W. Singer. "Effect of almonds on insulin secretion and insulin resistance in nondiabetic hyperlipidemic subjects: A randomized controlled crossover trial." *Metabolism* 57.7 (2008): 882–887.

bibliography and resources

Bibliography

Abhimanyu, G., MD. "Insulin Resistance in the Pathogenesis of Dyslipidemia." *Diabetes Care* 19.4 (April 1996): 387–389.

American Diabetes Association. "Nutrition Principles and Recommendations in Diabetes." *Diabetes Care* 27, Suppl. 1 (January 2004): 55.

Appel, L., MD; M. Brands; S. Daniels, MD; N. Karanja; P. Elmer; and F. Sacks, MD. "Dietary Approaches to Prevent and Treat Hypertension/A Scientific Statement From the American Heart Association." *Hypertension* 47 (2006): 296–308.

Benson G., R. Franzini Pereira, and J. Boucher. "Rationale for the Use of a Mediterranean Diet in Diabetes Management." *Diabetes Spectrum* 24 (2011): 36–40.

"CountingEveryStepYouTake."HarvardHealthLetter,September2009. *www.health.harvard.edu/newsletters/Harvard_Health_Letter/2009/ September/counting-every-step-you-take.*

Esposito, K., M. Maiorino, M. Petrizzo, G. Bellastella, and D. Giugliano. "The Effects of a Mediterranean Diet on Need for Diabetes Drugs and Remission of Newly Diagnosed Type 2 Diabetes: Follow-up of a Randomized Trial." *Diabetes Care* (2014): 1935–5548.

Hanley, A.J., A.J. Karter, K. Williams, A. Festa, R.B. D'Agostino Jr, L.E. Wagenknecht, and S.M. Haffner. "Prediction of type 2 diabetes mellitus with alternative definitions of the metabolic syndrome: The Insulin Resistance Atherosclerosis Study." *Circulation* 112.24 (August 2005): 3713–3721.

Katcher, H.I. "Dietary factors in relation to rheumatoid arthritis: A role for olive oil and cooked vegetables?" *American Journal of Clinical Nutrition* (January 2008).

Keijzers, G.B., B.E. De Galan, C.J. Tack, and P. Smits. "Caffeine can decrease insulin sensitivity in humans." *Diabetes Care* 25.2 (2002): 364–369.

Jenkins, D.J., C.W. Kendall, A. Marchie, A.R. Josse, T.H. Nguyen, D.A. Faulkner, K.G. Lapsley, and W. Singer. "Effect of almonds on insulin secretion and insulin resistance in non-diabetic hyperlipidemic subjects: A randomized controlled crossover trial." *Metabolism* 57.7 (2008): 882–887.

Larsson, S.C., and A. Wolk. "Magnesium intake and risk of type 2 diabetes: A meta-analysis." *Journal of Internal Medicine* 262.2 (August 2007): 208–214.

Linos, A., V. Kaklamani, E. Kaklamani, Y. Koumantaki, E. Giziaki, S. Papazoglou, and C. Mantzoros. "Dietary factors in relation to rheumatoid arthritis: A role for olive oil and cooked vegetables?" *American Journal of Clinical Nutrition* 70.6 (December 1999): 1077–1082.

Salas-Salvadó, J. "Reduction in the Incidence of Type 2 Diabetes with the Mediterranean Diet." *Diabetes Care* 34 (2011): 114–119.

"Vitamin D and Health." The Nutrition Source, a Website by the Harvard School of Public Health. *www.hsph.harvard.edu/nutritionsource/vitamin-d/*.

World Health Organization. "Draft Guideline: Sugars intake for adults and children." *www.who.int/nutrition/sugars_public_consultation/en/*.

Resources

Websites

USDA MyPlate.gov
www.choosemyplate.gov

Dietary Guidelines for Americans, 2010
www.health.gov/dietaryguidelines/2010.asp#tools

The Academy of Nutrition and Dietetics
www.eatright.org

American Diabetes Association
www.diabetes.org

U.S. Department of Health and Human Services Physical Activity Guidelines for Americans
www.health.gov/paguidelines

American Diabetes Association: Living with Type 2 Diabetes
www.diabetes.org/freeprogram

Harvard Health Publications, Harvard Medical School, Glycemic Index and Glycemic Load for 100-plus Foods
www.health.harvard.edu/glycemic

Whole Grains Council
http://wholegrainscouncil.org

U.S. Department of Health and Human Services National Institute of Diabetes, Digestive, and Kidney Diseases
www.niddk.nih.gov

American Diabetes Association Recipes for Healthy Living: Make Your Carbs Count!
www.diabetes.org/mfa-recipes/meal-plans

Diabetic Gourmet Diabetic Recipes
http://diabeticgourmet.com/recipes

Diabetic Living
www.diabeticlivingonline.com

National Diabetes Information Clearinghouse (NDIC) Directory of Diabetes Organizations
http://diabetes.niddk.nih.gov/resources/organizations.aspx

Dietitians (RD or RDN)/ Certified Diabetes Educators (CDE)

Janice Baker, MBA, RD, CDE, CNSC, BC-ADM
Registered Dietitian, Certified Diabetes Educator, Certified Nutrition Support Clinician, Board Certified-Advanced Diabetes Management
P: (619) 742-0145
Jbaker9@san.rr.com
www.bakernutrition.com
Facebook: *www.facebook.com/BakerNutrition*
Twitter: *www.twitter.com/JaniceBakerRD*

Michaela Ballmann, MS, RD, CLT

Registered Dietitian and Functional Nutrition Counselor
Founder, Wholify
Pasadena and Sierra Madre, CA
P: (626) 552-9355
michaela@wholify.com
www.wholify.com
Facebook: *www.facebook.com/wholify*
Twitter: *www.twitter.com/wholify*
Podcast: *www.wholify.com/nutritionally-speaking*

Andrea Chernus, MS, RD, CDE, CSSD

Registered Dietitian, Certified Diabetes Educator, Certified
Specialist in Sports Dietetics, Coauthor of *Nutrient Timing for
Peak Performance* (Human Kinetics, June 2010)
New York, NY
P: (212) 579-7070
arc@ChernusNutrition.com

Bonnie R. Giller, MS, RD, CDN, CDE

Registered Dietitian/Medical Nutrition Therapist, Certified
Diabetes Educator
BRG Dietetics & Nutrition, P.C., West Hempstead, NY
P: (516) 486-4569
bonnie@brghealth.com
www.brghealth.com
Facebook: *www.facebook.com/BRGDieteticsandNutritionPC*

Lise Gloede, RDN, CDE

Registered Dietitian/Nutritionist, Certified Diabetes Educator,
Owner, Nutrition Coaching, LLC, Arlington, VA 22207
P: (703) 516-4973
www.nutritioncoachlise.com

Jane Korsberg, MS,RDN,LD
Owner, Nutrition Reality LLC, Promoting Wellness &
Disease Prevention, Beachwood, OH
P: (440) 349-3873
F: (855) 430-9528
ohrdjane@gmail.com
Facebook: *www.facebook.com/NutritionRealityLLC*

Karen Marschel, RDN, LD, CDE
KM Nutrition Consulting, Inc.
www.kmnutrition.com
Karen@kmnutrition.com

Gita Patel, MS, RDN, CDE, LD, CLT
America's Vegetarian Diabetes Educator, Author, Consultant,
Speaker
gita@feedinghealth.com
www.feedinghealth.com

Hope Williams, RD, CDE
Certified Lactation Specialist, Wellcoaches, Trained Health
and Wellness Coach, Rhinelander, WI
P: (715) 499-1845
hopewilliamsrd@gmail.com

Lori Zanini, RD, CDE
Registered Dietitian and Certified Diabetes Educator,
Manhattan Beach, CA
P: (714) 627 5808
LoriZanini@gmail.com
www.lorizanini.com
Twitter: @LoriTheRD

index

about the author

Kimberly A. Tessmer, RDN, LD, is a published author and consulting dietitian in Brunswick, Ohio. A few of her most recent books include: *Your Nutrition Solution to Acid Reflux*, *Tell Me What To Eat If I Have Inflammatory Bowel Disease*, *Tell Me What to Eat If I Am Trying to Conceive*, *The Complete Idiot's Guide to the Mediterranean Diet*, and *Tell Me What to Eat If I Have Celiac Disease*.

Kim currently owns and operates Nutrition Focus (*www.nutrifocus.net*), a consulting company specializing in weight management, authoring, menu development, and other nutritional services. In addition, Kim acts as the RD on the board of directors for Lifestyles Technologies, Inc., a company that provides nutrition software solutions, developing a wide array of nutritionally sound meal templates.